Half My Size!

For someone who had all but given up on herself,
I found my way out of a lifetime of eating disorders.

I only had to change one thing...EVERYTHING!
I almost quit on myself, but I am so glad I didn't because you won't believe what's happening to me!

Foreword by Brenda Cacucci, M.D.

Contributions from Neil Wanee, M.D., John Aker, M.D.,
Muhammad T. Munir, M.D., and Matthew G. Newmann, A.C.S.M, C.P.T.

ROBANNE ROBIN

Copyright © 2012 Get Your STRONG On!, LLC

All rights reserved.

No part of this book may be used, reproduced, or transmitted in any manner whatsoever without the written permission of the Author. Printed in the United States of America.

For information address:
Get Your STRONG On!, LLC
P.O. Box 50985, Indianapolis, IN 46256-0985

ISBN 10: 0-988-57550-7
ISBN 13: 978-0-9885-7550-9

Photography by Luke Miller
Edited by Megan Corcoran

FIRST EDITION

For my Momma
...and every "fake skinny" or "300-pound me" out there
that dare not quit on themselves

Contents

FOREWORD

Brenda Cacucci, M. D.

Obesity is directly related to multiple health conditions: diabetes, high blood pressure, sleep apnea, reflux disease, cancer, heart disease, infertility, arthritis…the list goes on and on. Of equal importance is the impact of obesity on a person's quality of life. Many obese people are unable to find jobs, or suffer discrimination because of their weight. Some people are unable to participate in activities with their children and grandchildren. An obese person slowly becomes a bystander in his or her own life.

As a bariatric surgeon, I have the honor of helping a person achieve weight loss and ultimately seeing improvement or resolution of their health conditions. In addition, it is very gratifying to see a patient get their life back and begin enjoying it again. Bariatric surgery can be the "push" that helps them to succeed with weight loss.

However, it is very important for someone who is considering bariatric surgery to understand that there must be a commitment to a lifestyle change in order to be successful. I cannot stress enough that the surgery is just a "tool" to help a person lose weight. Unless there are changes in lifestyle regarding healthy eating, exercise and emotional health, the surgery will not work! Robanne has heard me say this over and over again. It is evident that she understands what she needs to do to be successful and maintain her weight loss. She will continue to fight her battle to remain healthy! I applaud Robanne for sharing her story about her lifelong struggle with weight. I have the pleasure of being able to share in her transformation from a person who felt as if she had no hope, to an amazing success story. I expect that people will be inspired by her story and find motivation to change their life for the better.

Dr. Brenda Cacucci is a bariatric and general surgeon in private practice at Meridian Surgical Group located in Carmel, Indiana. She attended Indiana University School of Medicine and completed her general surgery residency at St. John Hospital in Detroit, Michigan. She performs bariatric surgery in partnership with the St. Vincent Carmel Bariatric Center of Excellence, in Carmel, Indiana.

Neil R. Wanee, M.D.

As a family physician it is my job to meet patients where they are and hopefully find a way to motivate them to achieve better health through whatever path best suits that individual. For the morbidly obese (those more than 100 pounds overweight) it is often suggesting bariatric surgery. While it certainly is not without risk, when done by experienced surgeons it can be most effective in helping patients get a new lease on life. Most patients have exhausted other options by the time they are open to this. All they need is some encouragement and reassurance of the benefits. It is so wonderful to see people being able to move again and start to live a more normal life, often getting off numerous drugs. In Robanne's case, she not only decided to have the surgery, but after, dedicated her life to one of health and fitness. What a pleasure it is to have been a part of this dramatic metamorphosis. I applaud her dedication and am grateful for all the people she will encourage with her amazing story.

Dr. Neil Wanee is a board certified family physician currently practicing with St. Vincent Medical Group in Fishers, Indiana. He is a graduate of the Indiana University School of Medicine and completed his family medicine residency at Community Hospitals in Indianapolis, Indiana.

GLOSSARY OF TERMS
bazillion/cajillion (anything with an "illion" = a lot of dough $ (FYI bazillion is actually a word, who knew?)
chill + relax = chillax
crazy + amazing = kruh-mazing
expensive but ridiculous = expendiculous
expensive but necessary = expendecessary
expensive but worth it = expurthit
ridonculous = ridiculous but better
expensive + ridonculous = expendonculous (ok, I took it too far)
anything with an "F', effing, flipping, or freaking is exactly what you make it
holy crappits - like holy crap, but more fun
magnificent + fantastic = magnifitastic
nada enchilada = less than none, zilch, zero, absolute bupkis
padonka donk = large to the 10th power
pregenormancy = hall pass to pig out while pregnant
sister(s) = friend(s) -- I say "sister" a lot, but I'm talking to you too, brother
smart + sexy = smexy
squwenchy = like undies in a bunch but worse
terrific + wonderful = terrifical

Grammatically incorrect WORDS I OVERUSE:
All of the words listed above.

Other overused words/phrases:
"the sitch", the "situation" (no, not Jersey Shore style--don't worry), pump the brakes, just saying, grasshopper, freakish, YIPPEE!, REALLY!?, SERIOUSLY!?, hot mess, jacked up, anyhoo, kung-fu grip, sister(s), Splenda-coat

p.s. I love "air quotes" too.

Star Wars characters mentioned: YODA

Abbreviations:
AYFKM!!!! = are you freaking or flipping kidding me! (your call on the "F")
BTW = by the way
BFF = really...do I have to spell this one out for you?
HSF/HMF/HCF - Holy snikeys factor, holy crap factor, or holy moly factor (what is a "moly" anyway?)
MVM - minivan mom
NG - not good
OMG- oh my God
PT- personal trainer
STFD= shut the front door and if you want to be a fancy pants --STFFD = shut the front French doors
STHU = shut the "heck" up (eligible for an upgrade to its cousin STFU on certain days of the month)
What-evs = whatever
WTH - What the "heck", not be confused with its cousin "WTF"
YGG - you go girl (pronounced "gurrrl")

Fine Print: Direct & indirect references to Dr. Phil: a bunch.   References to Oprah: I lost count.
*DISCLAIMERS - My husband was not harmed in the making of this book...(well, maybe a little).

Half My Size!

1

Rah! Rah! Shish-Boom-Bah!

Why write a book? I mean, really, losing half my size after having bariatric surgery and getting my life back is way more than I ever dreamed (seriously). I had no idea I was going to lose 150 pounds and make this transformation. I think part of me really didn't think it was possible, or even if it was, that I would be able to do it. After all, I've spent my entire life as a walking eating disorder. But one day, I realized I am doing it. Holy crappits! I am doing it! I say it in the present tense because it is something I will work on everyday for as long as I breathe.

Anyhoo, I was reading an article last night about the fact that most people probably don't care about my story as much as I do. I get that. Because I am really not as kruh-mazing as I would like to think. What'd she just say? "Kruh-mazing," (pronounced cruh–maze-ing). It's my combo word for crazy + amazing, and heads up there are a lot more made-up words, as well as common texter abbreviations to come, (so don't bother trying to spell check this bad boy, and refer to the glossary of terms in the front of the book so you can keep up…from here on out, I am not going to help you). BTW, Google translate can't help you either, unless they speak Robanne.

I digress. I'd apologize, but I'm only going to do it again, so let's not cheapen it with an "I'm sorry." Back to the transformation. Big whoop-tee-doo. I had bariatric surgery and lost half my size. Mind you, it's a kruh-mazing accomplishment, but it's been done before. Here's the thing—It almost didn't happen and I want you to know why. I think back to that one day several years ago where one simple action changed everything for me. One seemingly tiny decision altered my course and made it possible for me to make long-term lifestyle changes. I didn't know it then, but I was so close to not making the right decision and ending up head-first in a ditch. Getting my butt up off that couch that day was the beginning of what would become an amazing 180º turn toward health and fitness. We'll get to all of that. Just know I had a major "make it or break it moment," and I was totally clueless at the time. Hindsight is always crystal (as in clear), and now I can see how I almost derailed myself.

So yes, I am beyond content with losing a padonka-donk butt-load of weight (literally). But, (there's always a "but") it wasn't exactly a straight line from A to Z. This story is about so much more than just losing the weight. It has to be when you've experienced childhood obesity, anorexia, bulimia, morbid obesity and bariatric surgery. This book is about yours truly... a work in progress that has been all over the hot mess spectrum in this life with weight, eating disorders, and body image. I dish up a lot of vulnerability here, so play nice, and, if you must talk trash...at least do it the good old fashioned way—behind my back.

Anyway, I was in too deep with my lifelong weight issues and depression, and thought for sure I was a goner. I had all but given up on myself, but somehow Map-quested my way out and found what I call my STRONG. That strength was there—strength I didn't even know I had. We all struggle with something, and I believe everyone has the ability to be strong in whatever area of their life that's got a hold of them (physically or otherwise). For you it may be losing 10 pounds. Wait a minute. We are a chunky-monkey nation...let's double that and say you could probably stand to shed a 20-spot? Or maybe you are like girlfriend over here and have a buck fifty to lose and bariatric surgery is part of your journey? Or just maybe you're jacked up with something else altogether? You fill in the blank. Regardless, what's hard is hard. And my friends, CHANGE is the mother of HARD. That's where the whole "getting my STRONG on" idea came from. Often in combination with professional help, anyone can get theirs on and inspire change in their lives no matter what the issue is. So I guess I'm writing this book to be that cheerleader. Rah! Rah! Shish-boom-bah! Hang on to your hats and glasses, keep your arms inside the ride, and buckle up friends...we're going in.

One more thing. I've only got one rule when you're reading this book. Here it is:

NEVER GIVE UP ON YOU. NEVER.

(as defined by Webster's)

inspire

to move or guide by divine influence; to move (someone) to act, create, or feel emotions: arouse; to cause something to be created or done

change

the act, process, or result of making or becoming different

strong

healthy; having powerful action or effect

2
300-Pound Me

August 02, 2009 – Journal entry

I am just two days away from having bariatric surgery which will change my stomach so I don't eat at as much and I will lose weight. It's called a laparoscopic roux en Y (pronounced roo-in-why). I have spent most of the last ten years eating pretty much anything I can get my hands on (king-size candy bars, diet soda, pasta, French bread, French fries, ice cream, cookies, cake...what-evs). I'm scared to death and the thought of giving up food is unimaginable. I am pretty much feeling like a human trashcan. I don't consume anything healthy. I am always tired and rely on others to get things for me, so I don't have to get up. It is hard to do anything that requires the bare minimum of physical effort. It's beyond ridiculous. I don't want to live this way anymore. Who am I kidding? I am not living; I am merely existing in skin that is suffocating me.

If gluttony's got an "A" game, well you're looking at it. Today, I did not get up until after 4 p.m. (other than to get food and return to bed to eat it—in bed!) If you count that as getting up, well then, I get up a lot. So basically, I had slept all night, woken up, eaten some waffles (in bed) with butter and syrup, and then slipped into a self-induced food coma for three more hours. Food is my drug, and it has been since my earliest memory.

It is now about 10:30 p.m., and I am going to go up to bed soon. Although, I dread having to huff and puff my B-hind up the stairs, so I may just pass out down here on the couch. My mind is racing. I am afraid of dying in surgery or having complications after. Truthfully, I'm afraid of just about everything. I need to get those fears out so I can hopefully move forward and do the next right thing. Seriously, at this point I'm eating myself to death daily, so what do I have to lose?

My nightly ritual involves cramming as much food down my throat as I can before I go to bed (pass out). I know Dr. Phil would say, "How's that working for ya?" It's not. Tomorrow I have to be on a clear liquid diet which hurts to even say. Since it's the day before surgery, it's required. Because I am so afraid of dying on the table, I'm going to have to do it. So on this last day of sheer gluttony, of course I'm gonna go out big—I mean eat like there's no tomorrow. BTW, part of me has been contemplating the idea of "no tomorrow" for years.

Tonight is different though. I tried to eat a big 'ol piece of cake, but I just couldn't do it. Food doesn't taste good anymore. Stuffing it down my throat doesn't work anymore. What started out as emotional eating, a.k.a. "comfort food," left the building with Elvis a long time ago. Food has gone from being my BFF to being my captor. I have been chasing comfort that hasn't been there for years. I guess it is sometimes easier to remain in the misery you know rather than make a change. Even if what you know is the painful reality of eating yourself into oblivion everyday to the point of passing out, only to wake up and do it all over again. Damn it. Why is change so scary? It's the uncertainty that freaks me out. What if I fail? God, I can't fail at one more attempt to lose weight. I just can't, but I don't know any other way to live. The food frenzy I've been in my entire life is finally over and I know it. It's paralyzing.

Food has always been there (except for the occasional sick day). Otherwise, it has perfect attendance... no nights, holidays, or weekends off. OH NO. Food is open 24/7. Best of all, it doesn't reject or judge me. It totally gets me. BTW, when you see a morbidly obese person and think, "OMG, why don't they get their sh@#! together and lose the weight?" just know they are so far ahead of you on that one. Every single day of my fat existence, there hasn't been a day that I haven't beaten myself up mentally. Not to be creepy or anything, but I often catch myself staring at skinny people in awe. They make it look so easy-peasy. How in the heck do they do it, and why can't I? I am so sick and tired of being sick and tired, I can't see straight. For years it has been the same stuff day in and day out. Saturated in my diseased thinking, I wake up, or "come to," depending on how you look at it. Somehow I claw my way out of the deep, dark abyss that has absorbed me, so I can trudge through the day. Yep...the D-word. If I dare admit it, I am severely depressed, drowning myself with each bite. I don't know how many hours during the last 10 years I have stayed in bed, buried under the covers to hide from myself.

I am tired of this slothful existence and I am beyond worn out. If it wasn't for this surgery, I don't know what I would do. I pray that I have the strength to do what I am told and follow all of the regimens I need to, to be successful. I am so desperate to have hope. I cling to the fact that I am heading for positive change. At least I hope so. I want to have a life...a healthy one. At least I have to believe that it is a possibility. Please, for the love of God...be a possibility. God grant me the serenity to accept the things I cannot change, the courage to change the things I can, and the wisdom to know the difference. Here we go...

Wait...there's one more thing—I lied about there only being one rule when reading this book. There's actually two. Here's the second one:

-WHEN YOU ARE BEHIND NEVER GIVE UP

WHEN YOU ARE AHEAD, NEVER LET UP-

That's **never** as in not ever; at no time; not to any extent or in any way

3

I WAS YOU

When I say I was you, I mean feelings-wise. I don't mean literally I was you. Our situations could be totally different, but our feelings eerily similar. If being morbidly obese is how you roll, then you may very well be like I was. In which case I am guessing, you are not in a good place. I'm talking NG. You are beyond overweight. It has gone well past just being fat. Food now controls you, tempts you, rules your every move. You likely plan your day around what you crave, what you will eat and when, and you make certain there is enough. At the grocery store, you take the walk of shame down the dessert aisle at some point each day so you are guaranteed to have enough sugar to tuck yourself in at night. You hide food from your family, even your kids, and your consumption is embarrassing. You are disgusted, and likely hate yourself, but you cannot stop.

Physically, mentally, emotionally, spiritually, and somewhat financially, you are a hot mess. You are tired all of the time, sweaty, short of breath with the slightest exertion, and your appearance is closer to that of a plus-size homeless Barbie than the woman your husband married so many years ago. If you're anything like I used to be…your blood pressure is high, your blood sugar is through the roof, and you have to look up the

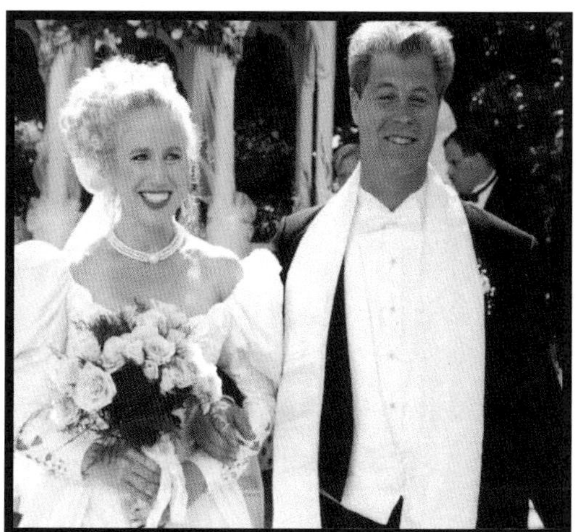

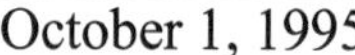

October 1, 1995

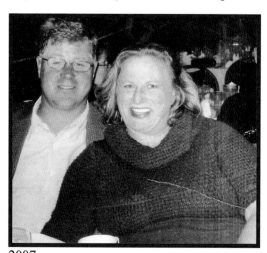

2007

meaning of "exercise" in Webster's. Your love life is non-existent and you pass out after meals only to wake up and stuff yourself with dessert. You sleep a lot, partially as an escape to try and hide and avoid your reality that reeks of gluttony. The sheer exhaustion of eating yourself silly is destroying you and your family, but yet you cannot stop. Depression is off the chain, but you'd rather ignore it and try and eat your way around it. You're sensitive and insecure, constantly seeking validation from others. You feel hopeless and lack direction. You are financially irresponsible and spending money is but another diversion that frequently gets you into trouble.

I've overused just about anything I can get my hands on – cigarettes, alcohol, shopping, money—pretty much everything except sex, drugs and gambling, (but I am pretty sure I'd be perfectly capable of that too). Truthfully, anything I have ever used and abused has been but a symptom of a deeper problem. Food has been no different. It's the hardest issue I have ever had to deal with. I have battled it every day of my life. It has never come easy for me, and I suspect it never will. It's not illegal and every social event on the planet is focused around it, (holidays, weddings, birthdays, baby showers, bar mitzvahs...geez-Louise...even funerals). There's no getting away from it! Probably in my coffin, there will be a Ho-Ho.

Food is my "drug of choice". It's another coping mechanism that I put to use from the get-go starting with childhood obesity, then anorexia, then bulimia, and morbid obesity. Talk about being messed up in the food department! I feel fortunate to have survived them all. Although I can't help but reference other issues, I want to focus on my struggles with food, my experience with bariatric surgery, and how I made the voyage from the couch to the treadmill. I just thought you should know I've got "other stuff" to deal with too (shocker). I am no rocket scientist, but I am pretty sure you don't get to be 300 pounds (or more) without stuffing down some big issues.

Losing weight, after bariatric surgery is only part of my story. Food kicked my padonka-donk butt! (I know I already used that term, but how many times do you get the chance to work it into a sentence? Padonka-donk! Padonka-donk! K, I'm good for a while). Anyway, the intricacies of weight and food issues are crazy-complex. I can't even begin to explain all of that psychology & physiology business. I can share my own experience with food addiction, and how I got my STRONG on to get where I am now. Bariatric surgery was the last house on the block so-to-speak, and therefore a major part of my story. First we'll talk about what led up to 300-pound me, but then I want to give you a glimpse through my eyes of what it's like to lose 150 pounds after bariatric surgery. I'm talking diet, exercise, excess skin, the plastic surgery that went horribly wrong, and the surgery to fix it…sex, shopping, clothes, you name it—it's all on the table.

BTW, in general, I am not for bariatric surgery or against it. Call me Switzerland, but it is an individual sitch-by-sitch decision, and my opinion doesn't mean jack when it comes to your life. So let's be clear, this book is by no means a recommendation or foretelling of what your experience, or anyone else's for that matter, will be. Your journey is your own. I know for me, when I was facing my own issues and decisions with bariatric surgery, I was hella-overwhelmed and unsure. It helped me to research and ask questions, then sit tight on those answers for a bit. I contemplated my own surgery for several years before I did it. Eventually, I came to a place of clarity, guided by that information, and I was able to make what I believe was the right decision for me. If you are in that boat – "The S.S. Morbid Obesity," – then I wish the same for you. This is <u>my</u> story about the course I traveled from childhood obesity to anorexia, to bulimia, to morbid obesity, to bariatric surgery and to STRONG. It is one of hope that has completely knocked my fuzzy socks off and kicked even my wildest expectations up a few notches. But, it almost didn't happen. Let me tell you, after the surgery there were many temptuously difficult moments trying to align my 2 ounce stomach with my 300-pound brain. My coping mechanism had been ripped from my kung-fu grip. I had to learn to deal, without going to food as my default comfort. (Sure thing. I'll get right on that).

I'm going to tell it to you straight, so listen up. Don't be fooled by bariatric surgery. It is smexy-seductive and can lure you into a false sense of control coupled with the glamour of rapid weight loss. But I assure you friends, those feelings are fleeting unless you make some serious changes. (That's "changes" with a capital "C"). If you are willing to make them, then please, have at it. This surgery can be an amazing tool to get your mojo moving in the right direction and help you begin to repair the damage. <u>But, it is not "the repair</u>." Write that down. I hope by sharing my own experience with you, it will help you find your way. Keep in mind I am by no means an expert on this matter, or anything really. There are some things to consider for sure, and consider them you must (I channel Yoda occasionally). But, just in case I start to sound like little Miss Know-it-all, keep in mind my surgery was just over three years ago since I have completed this book. So, I am not even smarter than a 5th grader at this point.

Having bariatric surgery was like walking the plank into a whole new way of living. Surgery or no surgery, there is no long-term weight loss success without making the lifestyle changes we've all heard about our entire lives. You know the ones I speak of…DIET & EXERCISE. For the bariatric patient, the post-operative diet is very specific and compliance is mandatory in order to achieve long-term success. By "mandatory" I mean, NOT OPTIONAL.

NEWS FLASH: Losing weight is hellaciously hard. PERIOD. There are no short-cuts for sale (that work) to get you there. I may be mistaken, but there seems to be a few rumors circulating that bariatric surgery is a cinch, the old quick fix-a-roo, akin to cheating and taking the easy way out. (Don't even get me started). At the risk of being repetitive (I'm going to go for it anyway), let me clear this one up...this method of weight loss is not the equivalent of hitting the easy button! No slam-dunk here, friends. Like any surgery, bariatric surgery is dangerous. Playing by the rules afterward is about as easy as, oh...I don't know, changing EVERYTHING about your lifelong patterns of self-destructive behavior. Go to a bariatric unit at any hospital and you'll see how "easy" it is not.

Worse than the rumors, are the assumptions made by people wanting to have this surgery. As I see it, bariatric surgery's top two claims to fame are #1 - that it will fix everything and, #2 - that exercise is optional. NO and NO. This is not the deal folks! Being non-compliant with the diet and exercise requirements can kill you. And if it doesn't kill you, it will certainly leave you in worse shape than you were before. Plain and simple, you cannot have the surgery and continue eating the foods you are forbidden to eat! And, you MUST, and I mean MUST, exercise! If bariatric surgery is even on your radar screen, don't take having it lightly. It's serious biz.

I have included pictures of my transformation in this book showing the before and after...and yes...we'll talk about the hanging skin and the reality of what's left after massive weight gain meets massive weight loss. And trust me friends, there is no topical cream or exercise that will get rid of what I am talking about. If I've missed it, Facebook me, K? For those of you considering bariatric surgery, or know someone who is, it's imperative to hear a few things. I have seen so much of the negative side of bariatric surgery, the people that don't succeed, the complications, and the bad rap this method of weight loss seems to get. I truly want to be an inspiration for bariatric peeps. This surgery can have remarkable outcomes if used correctly. I also want to combine that inspiration with a reality check of how serious this surgery is and the dedication it takes to have a shot at being successful (for more than five minutes). If there is anything I hope you will take away from this book, it would be that you only have to change one thing...EVERYTHING. If you are unwilling to change everything you are currently doing, then you should walk away now. SERIOUSLY. I'd say run, but if you are like I was, we both know that running ain't happening.

Maybe you'll take this drastic measure, maybe you won't. That's for you and your doctor to decide. Hopefully you will find that reading about someone who has been through it (and then some) to be helpful. It's a little harder to relate to information on weight loss of any kind from a skinny-mini who's never seen a fat day in their life. (Unless you are my doctor) I think talking to what I call "regular skinny" people about weight issues is just strange. By "regular skinny," I mean people who've never struggled with food and weight. I know it may seem alien, but they do exist. And if you are a "regular skinny," God bless you! But I'm not going to lie. "Regular skinnies" just don't get it, like some of us get it. They've never gone to some of the extremes I've gone to like throwing food away so I didn't eat it, only to get it out of trash later because I just couldn't resist it. Talk about putting a demoralizing spin on the five-second rule!

"Regular skinnies" have likely never stopped at multiple drive-thrus so they can get the double cheeseburger they want from here, and the burrito they want from there, only to eat it alone in their car so no one will see. They don't go to any lengths to satisfy food cravings. Way embarrassing, but I've done all of that and then some. Sharing these moments with you now is no longer shameful because I don't exist that way anymore. What an absolute miracle it is to say that today! After living so many years shrouded in secrecy, I am free. I betcha someone out there will read this and find they can relate to my insanity and know they are not alone. There's no shame in that friends.

Maybe you don't need to lose an ounce, but wouldn't mind borrowing a shred of hope during a hard time? This book is for you too, and any hope you find in these pages is yours to keep, sister. (I say "sister" a lot because that's how I roll. But just know I mean "brothers" too. Sometimes I throw in a gender neutral "friend". Just depends on how I want to say it. Nonetheless, sisters, brothers, friends--Kumbaya, I'm talking to all y'all).

Beyond that, I have a message to share with everyone, particularly the young bucks. It's not about being SKINNY. It's about being STRONG and fit. I guess you could say I'm pretty fired up about it. My passion has become inspiring anyone who struggles with food issues, body image, and lifestyle changes, starting with the kiddos. They need to know that STRONG is where it is at! So make sure you tell them. It's not about being a size double-zero toothpick, navigating their way through the skinny jean jungle. K? Don't get me wrong skinnies..."healthy skinny" is awesome...it's "fake skinny" I want kids to take a hard right from.

Today I can handle food for the first time in my life. By "handle" I mean I can manage nourishing my body and maintaining a healthy weight successfully one day at a time. By no means do I have this thing licked. I have a healthy fear of my food addiction and know all too well the mass destruction I am capable of. Heck, I ate an entire sheet cake once, and if I'm not careful, that insanity will repeat itself. Wait a minute. Back the truck up. Did she just say food addiction (again)? Yup yup. Am I calling you a food addict? Chillax. Nope, that's for you to determine. But, I happen to be one, and I have repeated this insanity over and over again my entire life. In case you need a refresher on the definition of INSANITY it means: "repeating the same patterns and expecting different results." YAY! So far it sounds like I am an insane food addict with a flair for the depressive side. Please continue.

Insanity - repeating the same patterns of behavior and expecting different results

It surely can't get any worse than insanity right? Oh yes it can sisters. At least with insanity there is the implication that you are expecting or hoping for a different outcome. So although insanity may sound like the bottom of the barrel, I assure you there is a trap door beneath it. That trap door my friends is indifference. When you hit this stretch of the highway…you pretty much could care less about yourself. That's the scariest road I've ever been on.

(Insert trap door here)

Indifference - not interested or concerned about something (namely yourself)

Just for Today

Just for today I will try to live through this day only, and not tackle all my problems at once. I can do something for twelve hours that would appall me if I felt that I had to keep it up for a lifetime.

Just for today I will be happy. Most folks are as happy as they make up their minds to be.

Just for today I will adjust myself to what is, and not try to adjust everything else to my desires. I will take my luck as it comes and fit myself into it.

Just for today I will try to strengthen my mind. I will study; I will learn something useful; I will not be a mental loafer; I will read something that requires effort, thought and concentration.

Just for today I will exercise my soul in three ways: I will do somebody a good turn and not get found out; if anybody knows of it, it will not count; I will do at least two things I don't want to do; just for exercise. I will not show anyone that my feelings are hurt; they may be hurt, but today I will not show it.

Just for today I will be agreeable. I will look as good as I can, dress becomingly, talk low, act courteously, criticize not one bit, not find fault with anything and not try to improve or regulate anybody except myself.

Just for today I will have a program. I may not follow it exactly, but I will have it. I will save myself from two pests: hurry & indecision.

Just for today I will have a quiet half hour all by myself and relax. During this half hour, sometime, I will try to get a better perspective on my life.

Just for today I will be unafraid. I will enjoy that which is beautiful and I will believe that as I give to the world, so the world will give to me.

*Just for today is prayer from an anonymous self-help program.
There are a few nuggets in there I like to remember on a daily basis.

4

Thunder Thighs

I'm pretty sure my struggle with food and weight began in the womb. It's certainly been the main attraction in my life going back as far as I can remember. And while there have been other issues for me to deal with I am only going to put snippets of my life in this book. The entire story is a whole 'nother Oprah, and for sure another book. I will add tidbits here and there to give a little background on the sitch, but the rest of my life's ribaldry we'll hang on to for a bit.

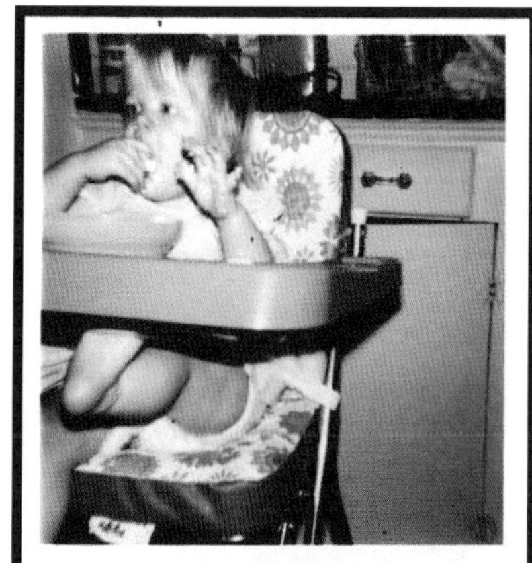

I grew up in Louisiana, well actually, no…I lived in Louisiana until my parents divorced when I was five years old. So, not exactly growing up there. Anyway, we lived on 55 acres of country bumpkin awesomeness. I had a horse named Goldie Locks (my own freaking horse). Living on a farm in the country, we weren't exactly pacesetters for healthy living. I can remember eating buttered white bread or a raw hot dog as a snack. Oohh...oohh and room temp Spaghetti-O's with meatballs right out of the can. We had fried okra and mashed potatoes with dinner all the time. I'm pretty sure that kind of eating came with Hee-Haw on in the background. Minnie Pearl, YGG! I don't know about your house, but I grew up under the effed-up wisdom of the "clean your plate" generation. That thinking screwed a lot of us up (thank you very much).

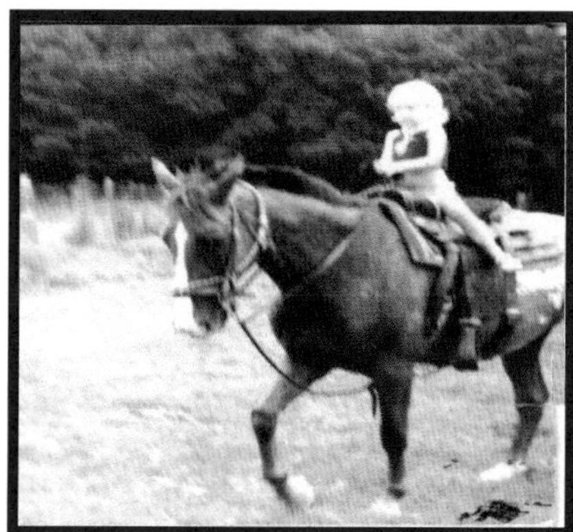

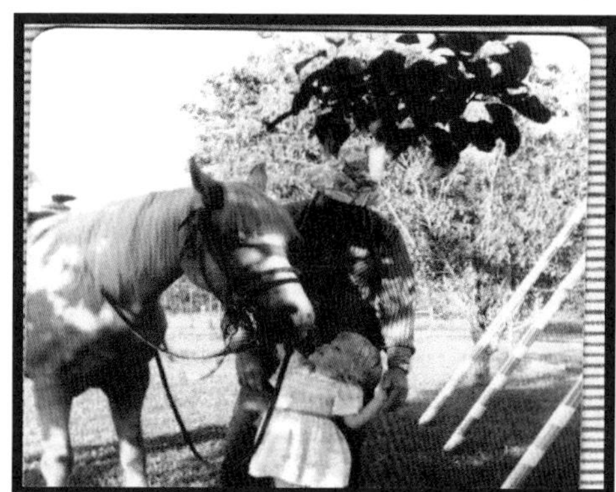

1972-1976'ish

Add that to the fact that I was naturally a chunky kiddo. Hang on a sec..."chunky?" WTH kind of description is that for a girl? Was I freaking salsa? Guess so. Anyway, salsa here could look at an apple and gain five pounds. Later I remember being called "thunder thighs" pretty much all through childhood. "Thunder thighs"…now that's what every girl dreams of being called (NOT). I managed to put it to good use though. It rocked as a tomboy playing tackle football with the boys. I was a force to be reckoned with in Michael Prowsey's back yard, which doubled as the neighborhood football field. It didn't take long for the boys to amend the general rule that a girl couldn't be tackled. Oh, no—I was fair game, but I still bulldozed right over them like a diesel Mack truck. Nine times out of ten I was first pick when we were choosing teams. My brother still needs therapy over that one. They nicknamed me "Riggins" after NFL Hall of Famer, fullback John Riggins of the Washington Redskins. Don't worry if you don't know who he is…doesn't matter. Just know I was one heck of a football player, and on Long Common Drive sports nicknames were earned and not handed out freely. I got to be called "Riggins." Me. I was the one everyone wanted on their team, and I was the only girl on the field. That's some serious street cred right there. Best of all, football made every ounce of my awkward, un-girlie, chunky, thunder thighs appearance vanish for four quarters.

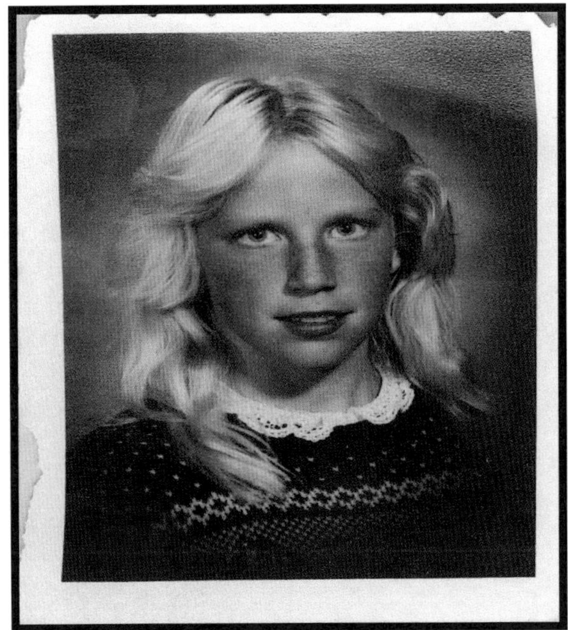

I'd rather be playing football than wearing this sweater.

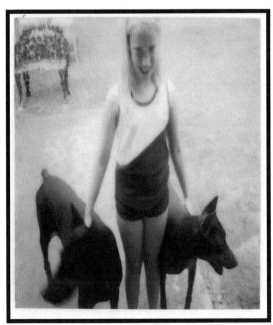

Chunky, thunder thighs, big-boned…AWESOME.

Then the unthinkable happened. Boobies developed and I was forced into early retirement. I had to cash in footballs for Barbies. Trading in my “Riggins” notoriety and cleats for some uncomfortable sparkly flats and a training bra wasn’t exactly my idea of a good time. But it seemed like the girlie-girl thing to do. I mean I guess I kind of wanted to be like the other girls, even though I had no clue where to start. They all had mad skills in the nail-painting and hair-doing departments. Me...well, not so much. Freaking detangling my hair was an all-day event, and once I tried to put on mascara and almost took my eye out. But, I desperately wanted to be pretty like my sisters and fit in with the other girls, so I kept at it. I wanted a boy to notice and be interested in me for something other than as a fullback. Fat chance.

I was always taller than the other girls and the boys too. Just when I thought it couldn’t get any worse than “chunky” or “thunder thighs”...it did. Since I weighed more, I was often referred to as “big boned.” WTH!...REALLY? Big boned? That’s a real charmer when describing oneself. That’s right up there with “you have child-bearing hips,” which was used to describe me several years later in life. Awesome.

So throw in some braces and acne and I’ve got all the self-esteem of a cumquat. I was always comparing me to you, trying to compete with how pretty you looked versus how inadequate I felt. Since you always looked better than I felt, it was always an unbalanced equation. *$E=mc^2$ ‘effed up. After I hung up my cleats, I was transparent to boys, and I sure as heck didn’t fit in with the girls. I mean, I wasn’t hideous or anything, but I wasn’t Bonne Bell, shiny, lip gloss cute either. I was just big enough to not be thin, which in junior high school might as well have made me Rotunda Splivitz. The boys never asked me to dances, and the girls just kind of tolerated me. I felt like I wasn’t good enough, and certainly not worthy of anything. Food really became my security blanket then. It did not judge me and it kept me company on a lot of Friday nights when my phone didn’t ring. So yeah, food and I became instant BFF’s.

CHUNKY...THUNDER THIGHS...BIG BONED...
CHILD BEARING HIPS...AWESOME.

*BTW, I know I am mocking the theory of relativity. $E=mc^2$ ‘effed up has no mathematical relevance to anything. But it sounds snazzy, so go with it. I told you not everyone speaks Robanne.

ROCKING THE CASBAH AND THE MID '80'S

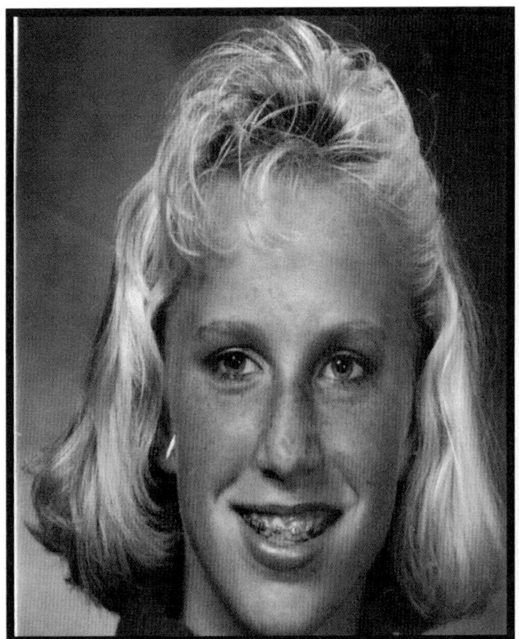

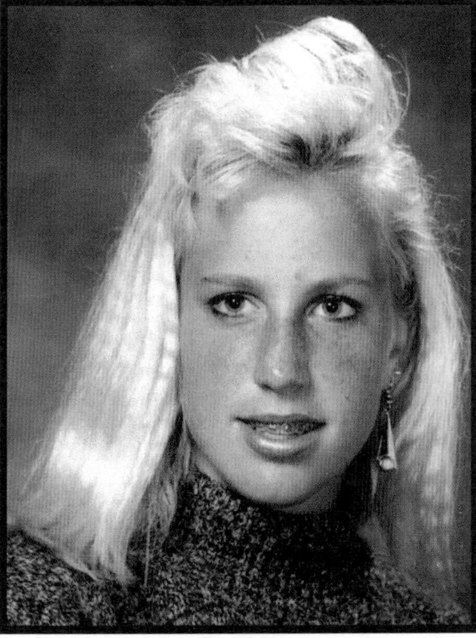

Hey…when you are done with my blue eye shadow, hand me my crimping iron and Aqua Net hairspray. Turn up the Duran Duran, and don't you dare spill anything on my Forenza sweater or jack up my Jordache jeans.

5

Fake Skinny

FOOD is an "F" word and I've felt out of control with it most of my life. Things really took a nose dive in my mid-teens, when for a while I flirted with anorexia. Definition of anorexia - I was going to get all clinical on you and put a whole sha-bang on this illness here but, that's not this book. It's a story, not a lecture. Suffice to say, *anorexia* <u>is when you don't freaking eat!</u> NG...really NG.

In high school I remember trying to survive on diet soda and gum for lunch. Then, I went through a rice cake phase, which is basically like eating crunchy air. I was light-headed all of the time and felt like I was going to pass out. BTW, they call that low blood sugar, and that, friends, can put you in a diabetic coma, and punch your lights out—as in, GAME OVER. I would obsess about food and want to eat it so badly, but couldn't for fear of gaining weight. I had to "pretend eat" at group meals. I clanked my fork back and forth a lot to move food around. I figured if I wasn't just sitting there, no one would notice I wasn't actually eating. I would take the smallest bite I could, just in case I had to swallow it. If I could sneak it, I would even spit food out in my napkin. When the coast was clear, I would use the ol' napkin again to smuggle out the larger chunks. I loved me some napkins. As time went on, it became clear that I wasn't a very "good" anorexic. Between the starving to death, constantly wanting to pass out, and the meal-time shenanigans, I had to throw up the white napkin, so I could literally begin throwing up.

Since I "failed" at anorexia, I started my love/hate relationship with bulimia. *Bulimia* (technical definition): <u>eating and barfing, or eating, barfing, and over-exercising to compensate for all the eating</u>. NG to the 10th power. I could eat massive amounts of food and then throw it all right back up. Scarf and barf. It was my big secret. I always had to "go to the bathroom" right after eating to purge. "Purge," that's a tidy way of saying "puke your guts out on purpose." I had to make sure I drank a ton of fluid when I was eating so afterward I could make myself gag and then watch all of this nasty food come flying back up. Lovely. If I didn't drink enough fluid, the food was too thick and got stuck coming back up. Yummy. I know, right. Imagine me bending over the toilet just hurling and trying not to get a rebound splash of toilet water on my face. Each time after I was done, I would do a spot check in the mirror to make sure my face wasn't too puffy and reddened, and that I didn't burst a capillary in my eye. This easily went on for several years. I tried not to forget to check the underside of the toilet seat too, because there was always barf on there (and that's a dead giveaway that you're a puker). BTW, it is a huge red flag if you know someone who high-tails it to the bathroom right after every meal.

Completely disgusting (I know). Funny thing about barfing up all of that stomach acid…it can completely destroy the lining of your esophagus and the enamel on your teeth. I guess I got lucky, my esophagus seems to be fine, but I had to have several teeth extracted followed by 14 root canals to repair all the destruction that barfing did to my teeth. For years there wasn't a day that went by that I didn't make myself throw up. I remember looking in the mirror and my hollow reflection staring back at me. But I was skinny damn it.

During this period of my life, I was what I call "fake skinny," because I could only be thin by actively practicing anorexia or bulimia. Please, pretty please, let's be clear... If what I've told you made it sound too glamorous, let me assure you "fake skinny" sucks. Although I'm pretty sure those closest to me had their suspicions, I have never told anyone all of that, not even the Mister.

Meet fake skinny. She's smiling on the outside, but dying like Starvin' Marvin on the inside.

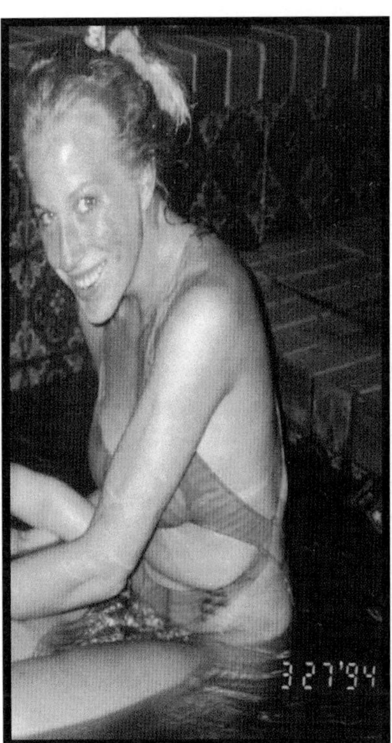

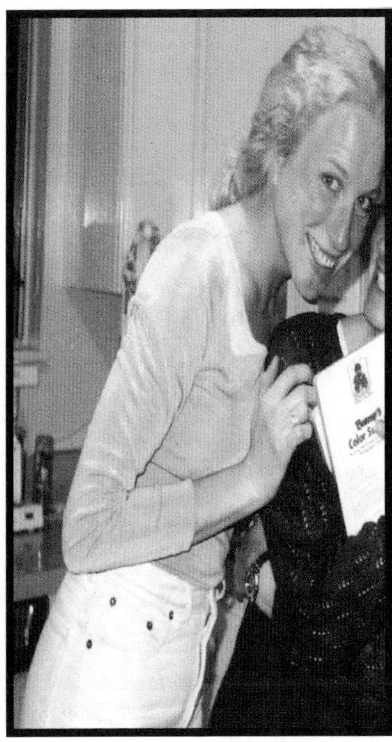

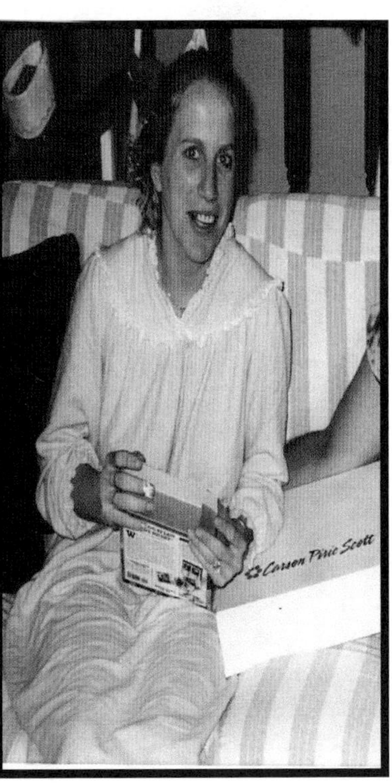

After several years of forcibly making myself vomit, bulimia had become far too exhausting. I couldn't take it anymore and I was running out of teeth. So one day I quit. I just kept binging without purging and voila…it didn't take long to enter the cage of morbid obesity that I kept myself in for the following decade. I overate to cope and probably to compensate for starving myself and scarfing and barfing for so many freaking years.

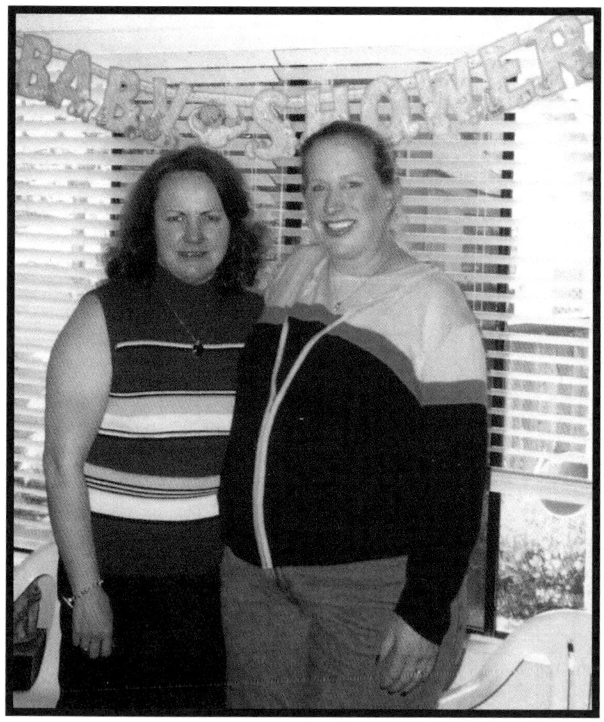

With my Aunt Diana during one of my "pregenormancies"

Along the way, I had three healthy babies. There was weight gain with each pregnancy, and after each child, I never lost all of the previously gained weight. Instead, I just kept adding to it. This "stacking" continued and by the birth of my third child, I was easily pushing 290. Motherhood is a total blessing and I am beyond grateful to be a parent. I don't blame being prego for my weight gain. Au contraire mon frère, I purposely used it as a hall pass to eat whatever I freaking wanted, whenever I wanted. Although I was certainly a volunteer here, and not a victim, the weight gain from each of these "pregenormancies" was difficult for me and I could not seem to find my way back. Instead, I was lost in the feelings of inadequacy of being a mother of three young whippersnappers. Eating a pint of ice cream each night (when I wasn't eating a sheet cake) allowed me to mentally check out from mothering young children. It made it a little more tolerable to be me, and let's just say I hated me.

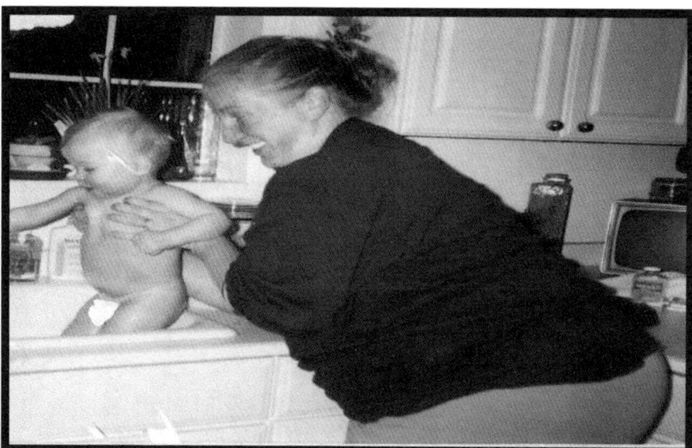
Baby's got back. And so does his momma.

I was consumed and overwhelmed with the care of my children and the demands of being mommy, worker bee, wifey, etc. It was too much for this puppy to handle. Some days, it was a major accomplishment just to get to unload the dishwasher and have a chance to take a shower. I didn't make time for me, EVER. Basically, in my mind, I was taking one for the team. That's what a good mom does, right? A good mom is supposed to put her children first, which in my case wasn't a stretch since I didn't take care of myself anyway. So being the overrun minivan mom (MVM) was a natural fit for me (although I'm pretty sure I was driving a Toyota Tercel or something). Quite frankly, it was just easier to completely let myself go – and I mean A-wall, off the grid…I'm talking underground, let myself go. Little did I know, I was saying Adios, sister! See you in a decade.

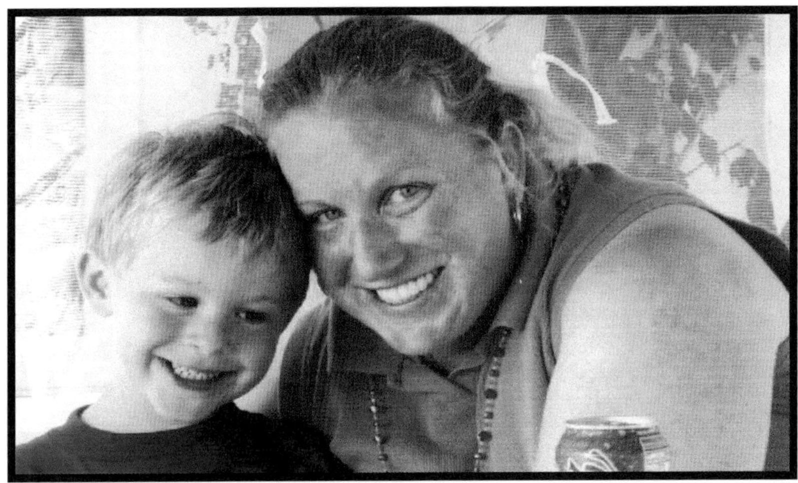

During that 10-year span of my morbid obesity (1999-2009), I was a jacked-up, hot mess. Food consumed me. It swallowed me whole (when I wasn't swallowing it). I was always planning my next food frenzy, which was daily. I didn't exercise and wasn't able to participate actively with my children. I was benched on the sidelines of life watching and wishing I could join in. At the park I sat down and watched the kids play. As Dr. Cacucci has said, I was "a bystander in my own life". I could not run around and play chase. Heck, I could barely even climb the stairs in our house.

At the pool, I sat on a lawn chair fully clothed. I would rarely put on a bathing suit or go into the water. Somehow I did manage to scrounge up two photos of me in a swimsuit during that decade. I must have lost a bet or something. Anyhoo, if you've ever gone to a public swimming pool and you know you are the fattest person there, or at least rounding out the top five, it literally feels like you are under a microscope. I was always consumed by what I presumed people thought about me. I'm really not sure why I cared because anything others were thinking was no match for the shots I took at myself. The meanest person on the planet couldn't hold a candle to my own self-deprecating inner dialogue.

The incredible amount of energy and the Herculean effort it took to plan all of those food binges was exhausting. Like Dr. Phil would say… " it takes a lot of work to be that overweight". He's more than right. It was a full-time, 24/7 operation in which I planned, plotted and schemed my binges from the moment I woke up, until the minute I passed out. Each year of that decade felt like a dog year. I felt so ugly, so fat, and so unkempt all the time. I couldn't seem to get anything going to get my groove back. Honestly, I never really had a groove in the first place (but you can't blame a girl for wanting one).

Food as you know was my BFF and did not like to share me with anyone else. Over the years, it totally took over. It decided everything...what I did or did not do. I neglected my family because I had to feed my addiction that had a kung-fu grip on me. My favorite "escape meal" was spaghetti. We ate it at least twice a week. And man...could I put some back. A meal usually consisted of two giant plates full of spaghetti with garlic bread...and of course dessert later. My other beloved faves were biscuits and gravy and just about all fast food (especially French fries). I would eat like gangbusters, well past the point of being full. Like a trooper, I would keep on eating because it tasted and smelled good, and heck—because it was there (and I could reach it). I didn't want to waste it (good plan). Growing up, I remember hearing "don't put it on your plate unless you're going to eat it." So what's a girl to do? It was on my plate (because I put it there), so I followed the clean-your-plate prescription, and I ate it. At this point in my life, I knew better than to follow those instructions, but I did it anyway.

In addition to being an "F" word, food is also a sneaky bastard. For the most part, it is an acceptable addiction. I mean it's not like it's a crack pipe or anything. You're not going to get arrested for eating an entire sheet cake. Even though I knew the danger I was flirting with, I hid behind the fact that food was permissible to go overboard with (and overboard without a life raft I went). Once I did, I felt any sense of control over my life slip through my finger tips. I was really screwed. I had an acceptable addiction to food with an unacceptable outcome of being 300 pounds.

FOOD...CAN'T LIVE WITH IT, CAN'T LIVE WITHOUT IT (PERFECT)

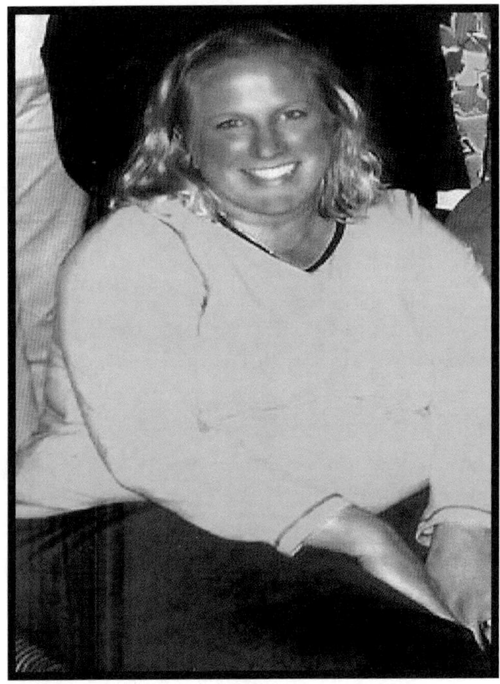

This picture was part of a group photo at a girl's night out sometime between 2006-2008. I'm not the best historian when it comes to pictures of 300-pound me. That's because I destroyed any pictures of me that I found. The camera may add 10 pounds, but it sure as heck doesn't add 150! I didn't want to have photos of myself that would remind me how out of control I was with food.

YOU CAN'T CHANGE WHAT YOU DON'T ACKNOWLEDGE

—DR. PHIL

6

Really Buddy?

What happened to me? I'll tell you what happened. I had to hit rock bottom sisters. For me that involved having the snot scared out of me, not once, but twice. In a nutshell, I had to go to the ER twice within a four month period. My resting heart rate the first trip was 201, and 206 on the second. If you've ever experienced this, it literally feels like a jackhammer in your chest. It stopped me dead in my tracks both times. Yeah, I know. I'm not the sharpest tack in the pack, so it took two roundtrip tickets to the ER for me to take notice. The first encounter was like getting a speeding ticket. You might slow down for a couple of weeks after you get one, but then you're right back at it. However, after the second ER visit, I knew I was facing some serious health jail time. I remember lying there on that cold, hard slab of a bed in a room that might as well have been on another planet. I felt so far away...so out of control. At age 37, I caught a glimpse of what morbid obesity had in store for me. NG.

What essentially was my own doing scared the ba-jeezus out of me! Thank God it did, because I don't know that I would have made a change otherwise. I was already on Metformin, a drug for my high blood sugar, and blood pressure meds were coming soon. I was constantly short of breath and sweaty without much effort. Up until that point, none of those things were enough to get me to change. But somehow, lying there alone in that sterile room, I knew my covers had been pulled BIG TIME. My obesity could no longer be ignored, and I had been ousted right on out of my 300-pound closet.

I had tried every diet out there during that 10-year period with no success. More accurately, I deprived myself off and on under the guise of a calling it a diet, but I was never able to maintain it, and I never changed my lifestyle. In fact, after so many repeated failures, I became frustrated in a millisecond. If I didn't see immediate results, I just quit. I was scared to death of having bariatric surgery, but now after all the ER biz, I was more scared not to. In early 2009, I went to see my primary care physician for a sinus infection and we began talking about my weight. I was petrified to discuss bariatric surgery with him, thinking he would judge me. However, I knew I could not leave his office without seeking some advice. This doctor was instrumental in helping me to consider bariatric surgery as a serious option for me. Rather than condemn this method of weight loss, he supported it as a helpful tool for the morbidly obese. He shared with me that he knew of several patients who had lost considerable amounts of weight and were living full, healthy lives as a result. I needed every bit of direction and encouragement he offered me that day.

Thank you, Dr. Neil Wanee, for guiding one heck of a lost soul and pointing me back in the direction of hope. I had forgotten that hope was still on the map. Thanks for the reminder.

hope - a chance or likelihood for something desired, something wished for

It was then that I began the process of seeking approval through my health insurance for bariatric surgery. It required about six months of pre-operative testing with lab work, EKG's, echocardiograms and stress tests, a sleep apnea screening, bariatric education classes, meeting with a psychiatrist as well as a dietician. There were probably other requirements too, but you get the gist.

Part of my pre-operative work involved recounting all of the diets I've tried in my life. Here's an interesting stroll down Weight Gain Lane. I had to go through and think of all the times I dieted, and what precipitated the weight gain. Talk about the assignment from hell! I mean who wants to recap a lifetime of failures? Now it was time to swallow some serious chunks of truth about myself, so I did it. This was a very insightful experience as I had never looked back at the sequence of events in my life in terms of when I gained weight and why. Along with anorexia and bulimia completely messing up my metabolism, there were some life events that sent me into a food tail spin. There was a job loss that crushed my identity and a miscarriage before my first child was born that rocked my world. I also quit smoking when I got pregnant which was good for at least 25 pounds. Add all of that up, plus the three pregenormancies I told you about, and by my math I come up with 300 pounds. Honestly, I can't believe I didn't weigh more.

If I think about all of the diets I have tried in the past, none of them (as you may have guessed) worked for more than five, maybe ten minutes tops. Let's see…not to single out any one diet, I'll rip on a bunch of them that I have tried…cabbage soup something or other, some random cookie diet (they'll try anything in Hollywood), no carbs, low carbs, no simple carbs, only whole grain carbs, and OMG the dreaded meal replacement shake! I'm not a shake hater or anything. In fact, certain shakes are awesome and I use them all the time now, but in addition to meals, not instead of. Big diff. Then there was no white flour or sugar, and not eating after 6 p.m. Dare I mention the "fat-free" movement? (I'm pretty sure we all got fatter). I've been a vegetarian, I've vegan'd, and I've gone gluten free. BTW, vegans, veggies and sans glutens out there...you are some of the healthiest people I know, so I'm not knocking you. It just didn't work for me because I wasn't in it for anything other than my pursuit of "fake skinny." I have also gone the support group route and the pay-by-the-pound weight loss programs, none of which worked long-term for me. The point is, if you are anything like me, you've tried a few things to lose weight. Some good in theory, some, well...not so much. If you are as fortunate as me, all you have to show for your dieting endeavors is losing weight for about half a second, followed by regaining it all back along with a few extra bonus pounds. YIPPEE!

This pattern of repeated failures further plunged my self esteem into the previously barfed in toilet, and my feelings of hopelessness and depression did a Mt. St. Helens. This is when the eating really got out of control. Indifference had arrived. I had given up, convinced nothing worked…basically FORGET it. FORGET me.

FORGET having any hope. I really, truly believed there was no way out of this existence and I would be stuck as 300-pound me forever.

After recounting all of my dieting disasters on paper, I had to go see a psychiatrist and talk about "my stuff". Oh goodie gumdrops. I was nervous, I mean who wants to be called to the mat and talk about why they are the way they are? I was wondering what questions he would ask me, and how I would respond. This was a crucial meeting because insurance approval for my surgery hinged upon this guy's sign-off on my mental readiness to have it. Me and mental readiness…oh boy.

I went in and prepared myself for the big inquisition. I just wanted to get it over with and say what he wanted to hear so he would put his John Hancock on my paperwork. I took a seat trying not to look too nervous, being sure to keep my arms pressed firmly to my sides to conceal the circles of perspiration underneath each armpit. He proceeded to ask me, "Do you think you have a problem with food?" I'm pretty sure I had to keep my eyeballs from popping out of my head when I heard that. What kind of freaking question is that to ask a morbidly obese person? That's kind of like asking an alcoholic if they have a drinking problem. I was thinking... "Um...hello! I'm like 300 pounds over here. Heck yeah I have a problem with food!"

To say why I or anyone else gains weight is beyond my pay grade (way beyond). Even though, at times, I have proven myself not to be the brightest bulb on the tree, I'm pretty sure it's safe to say that eating is very emotionally soothing, and food is addictive (duh). It is but a symptom of a greater problem. So when the shrink asked me if I thought I had a problem with food, I was thinking—really buddy? Call me crazy, but I guess I thought food was a given in the "I have a problem with" section. Yeah, that box was checked alright. I know he had to ask, I guess to make sure my expectations were in line with the reality that awaited me. I took a deep breath and looked him smack dab between the eyes and said, "If I didn't have a problem with food, would I really be sitting here right now talking to you?" That was the truth, and apparently the right answer. $120 later I was cleared for take-off.

-LITTLE DID I KNOW THAT IN THE DARKEST MOMENTS

WHEN MY LIFE WAS SEEMINGLY FALLING APART

IT WAS ACTUALLY ABOUT TO FALL TOGETHER-

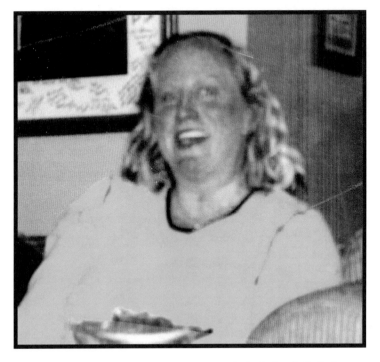

SOMETIME BETWEEN 2006-2008

(obviously not the best quality photo, but I'm holding a freaking piece of pie or something, so it made the cut)

AWARENESS WITHOUT ACTION IS WORTHLESS

—DR. PHIL

HERE'S A VISUAL FOR YOU ON HOW MUCH EXTRA WEIGHT I HAULED AROUND FOR 10 YEARS

300 POUNDS OF ME VS. 150 POUNDS OF STRONG

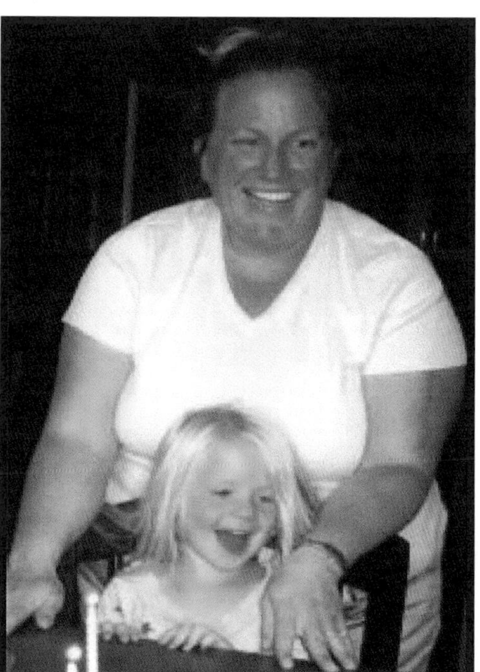

Walking around with an extra 150 pounds

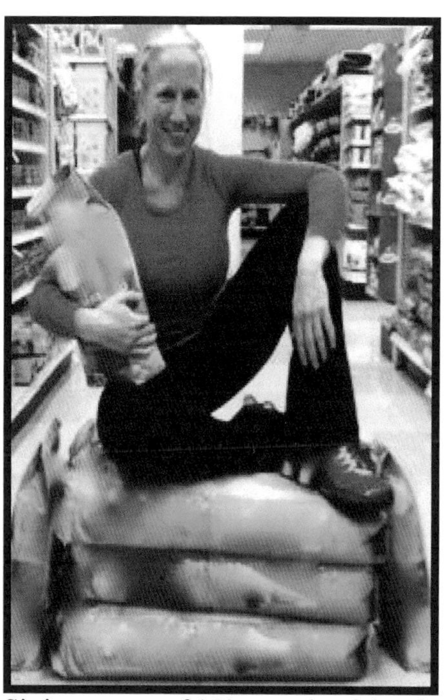

Sitting on top of 150 pounds of dog food

(MUCH EASIER TO SIT ON TOP OF THE DOG FOOD AS OPPOSED TO CARRYING IT AROUND)

Mother's Day 2003

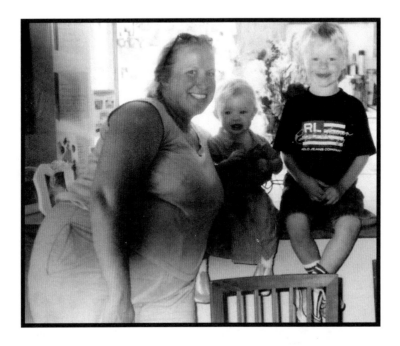

It's interesting to look back on myself at 300 pounds. Although I knew I was overweight during this decade, I had no idea I was *this* overweight (if that makes any sense). Funny thing is, in this photo, I am pretty sure I was sucking it in and trying to look as svelte as a big girl can.

What would you do if you knew you could not fail?

—John B. Sedgwick

Mother's Day 2012

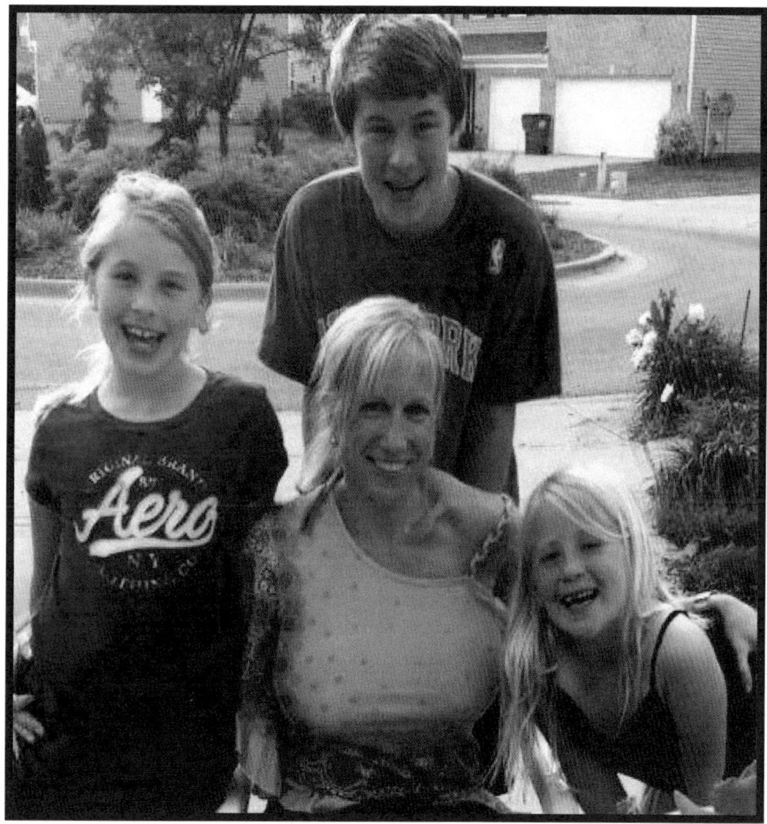

Leah age 10, Davis age 13, Halle age 8

Today, caring for my children begins with caring for myself

Although I was a good mom when I was obese, I can physically keep up with these whippersnappers now. This has proven to be quite helpful with one teenage boy and two preteen divas, I mean daughters. I can outrun every last one of them. Boo-yah!

AUGUST 2006

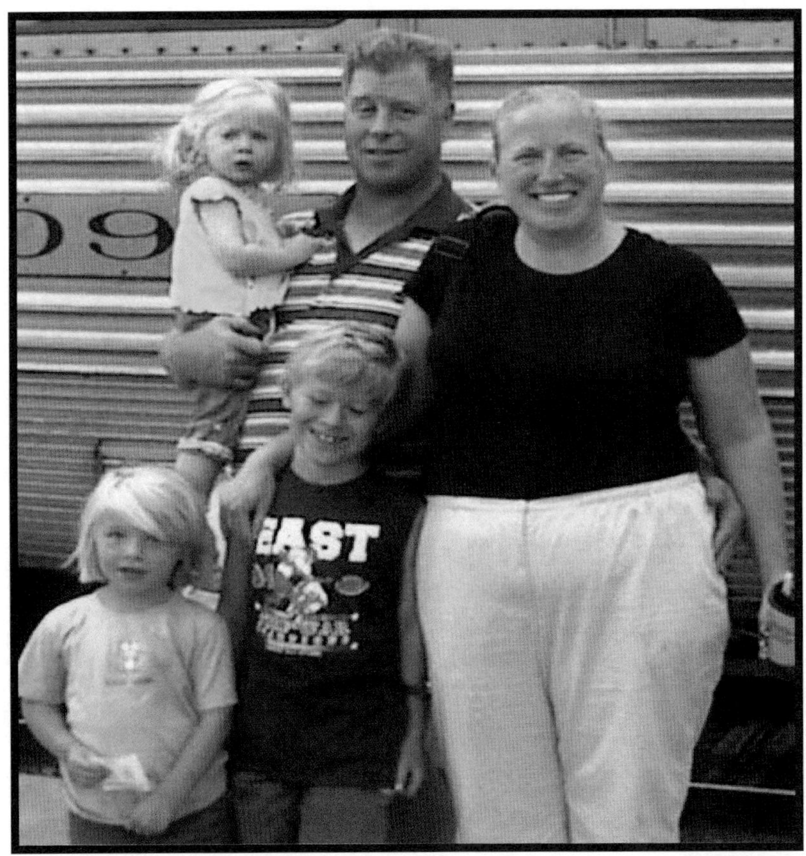

PAIN IS TEMPORARY, QUITTING LASTS FOREVER

—LANCE ARMSTRONG

FAMILY

AUGUST 2010

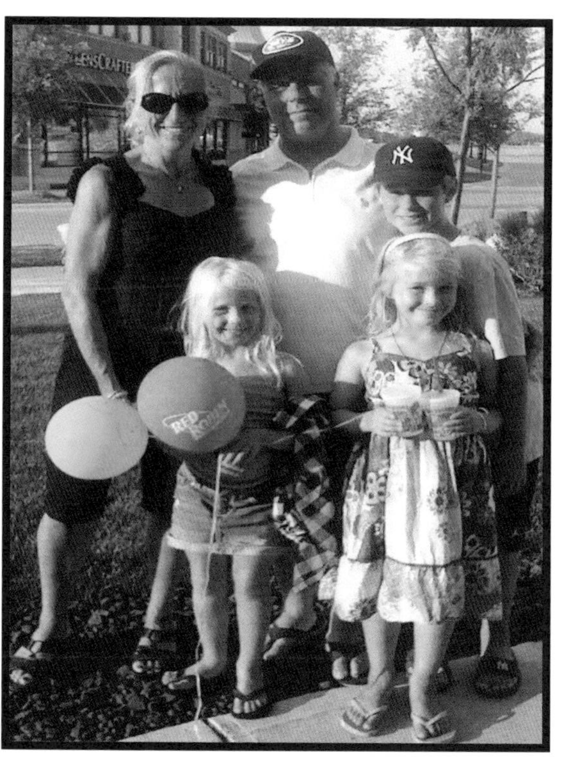

OCTOBER 2011

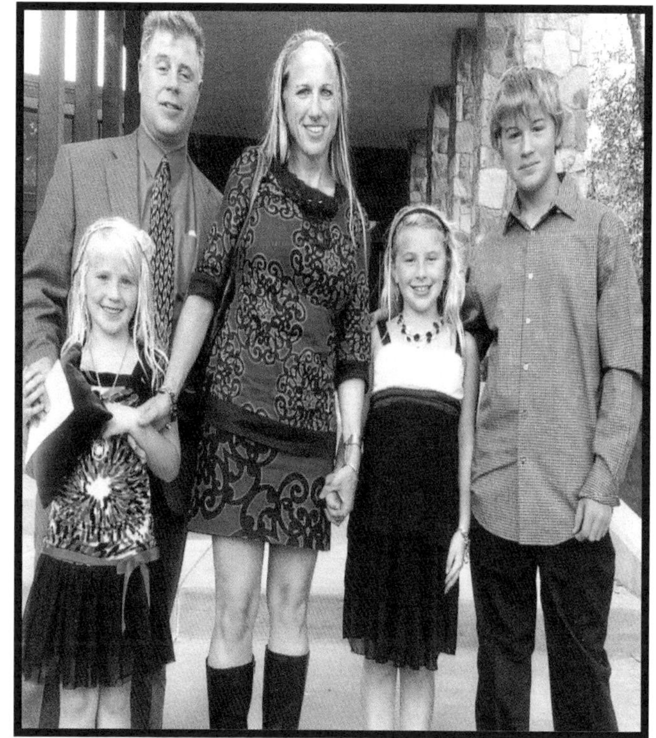

DON'T BE AFRAID TO FIND OUT HOW GOOD YOU CAN BE

IMPOSSIBLE = I'M POSSIBLE

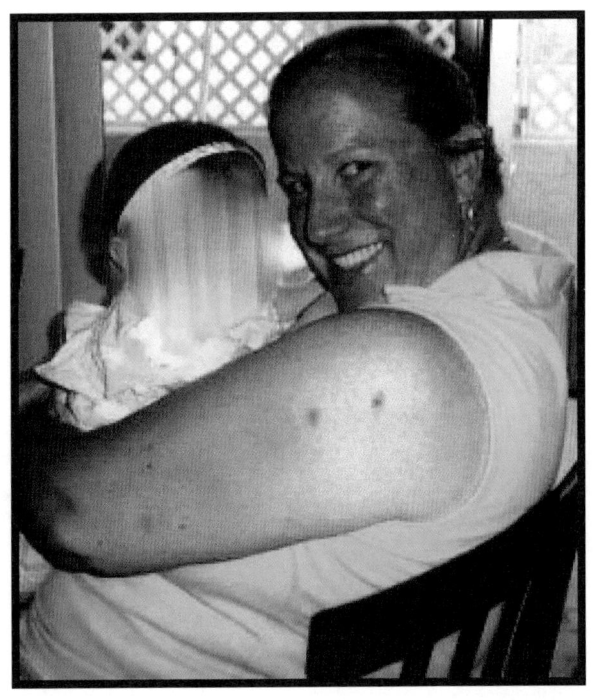

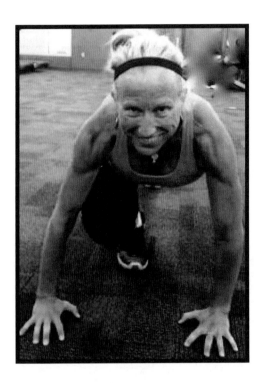

ON YOUR MARK, GET SET...GO FOR IT!

7

Cleared for Take-Off

There are many types of bariatric surgeries; roux-en-y, lap band, gastric sleeve...just to name a few. They are all different in the way they change anatomy, their mechanism of action, projected weight loss, lifetime dietary and nutritional modifications that are required, and potential complications. That's all well beyond the scope of this book, and quite frankly BOR-ing. Plus, last time I checked, it doesn't say M.D. after my name. The point is, there are many types of bariatric procedures. Google them, get enough on-line information to be dangerous, and then go chat with a real, live, human doctor.

Fast forward to August 4, 2009. On that date, I had a laparoscopic roux en y gastric bypass surgery.

Roux-en-Y

[ro͞o′ en wī′, ro͞o′änēgrek′]

Etymology: César Roux, Swiss surgeon, 1857-1926

a treatment for morbid obesity consisting of surgical division of the small intestine to form two arms; the jejunum is anastomosed to a gastric pouch and the bypassed duodenum connects the pylorus with an end-to-side anastomosis into the lower jejunum. Mosby's Medical Dictionary, 8th edition. © 2009, Elsevier

English translation: it changes the stomach and small intestine to cause weight loss by restricting food intake. It creates a small pouch to serve as the stomach, so you cannot eat as much making the body unable to absorb as many calories from the food.

Since that time, I have gone from 300 pounds to my current weight of 150, which I have been at for over a year and a half now. I made a 180 degree turn, going from hopeless to healthy. In essence, I did a 180 after losing 150. Utterly kruh-mazing, but this transformation has not been without its struggles and two tons of work. I said it earlier (but it bears repeating), there is no surgery, no quick fix, no magic pill or meal-replacement shake that will work (for more than five minutes) without making lifestyle changes. I only had to change one thing...EVERYTHING! How in the world do you do that you ask?

I had to "act" my way into better thinking rather than rely on my thinking to get my actions in line. I know from previous experience with other issues I have faced, changing self-destructive behavior doesn't happen by merely thinking about it. This is no different. Just because I had a surgical procedure that made my stomach smaller, I was still left with my "obese thinking," and therefore the accompanying bad habits that got me there in the first place. Making lifestyle changes has been completely backward for me. Before the surgery, I never once thought, "YIPPEE...let's go to the gym!" Since the surgery, whether I felt like it or not, I have had to consciously take the action of getting my butt up off the couch and go to the gym. If I didn't want to go...guess what?...I went anyway. It is actions like that which have proven to be lifestyle changers for me. Actions had to change first and the thinking followed later. Bizarre, but true. I ALWAYS remember that my best thinking got me to 300 pounds, not my best actions. It stands to reason then that my best thinking won't get me out of being 3-hundy!

I had to act my way out of my 300-pound thinking; first with food, and then with exercise. (I like a challenge apparently). This was not easy to take on for someone with the self esteem of a gnat on anti-depressants. It was time to get real and stop the Splenda-coating. This was life and death for me, and recess was over. In order to keep myself honest I would frequently remind 300-pound me of a few things. Here's a little "note to self" I put up on my bathroom mirror:

> Dear Robanne:
>
> You may not know what to do, but you sure as heck know what not to do. And if you forget what not to do, do the opposite of what you used to do. One more thing, I don't give a you-know-what if you don't want to go exercise or eat right. You already know what you need to do. So do it. Good talk.
>
> Love,
>
> Your body

Bottom line: it really doesn't matter if I want to play by the rules or not. I just do. Especially on the days I am dragging, I cheer myself on like this: No matter how slow I go, I'm still lapping the guy on the couch…(Just saying). So...OFF THE COUCH I MUST GET (thanks Yoda).

NOTE TO SELF:

MY BEST THINKING GOT ME TO 300 POUNDS, NOT MY BEST ACTIONS

NO MATTER HOW SLOW YOU GO, YOU'RE STILL LAPPING THE GUY ON THE COUCH

8

FOODIE

From one foodie to another—let's talk shop, shall we? There is no diet alone, on its own merit, that works. There just isn't. I think I would have found it by now if there was. So, duh…a post-op bariatric diet is no different. It is yet another type of diet. Well then, if I truly believe what I just said about diets, then merely following the diet plan won't work long-term. There has to be more, and there is. We'll get to that.

So now that I have a 2 ounce "pouch" (it's what they call the part of my stomach I use), what do I eat? To put it into perspective, right after surgery my stomach was roughly the size of a newborn baby's. I'll never forget when they brought me my first meal tray after surgery. It had one of those plates with a dome lid on it. The lady who delivered it said, "here's your lunch," and she removed the dome lid. What I saw before me was mind-blowing. On this plate staring back at me were two, tiny 30 ml cups, like the kind you pour cold medicine into. BTW, if you're not a metrics girl, 30 ml's = 1 ounce. Anyway, one of the cups had chicken broth in it and the other had grape juice. I was thinking—"You call that lunch? Shut the front French doors lady, that's not lunch!" Remember, you are talking to a girl who could put back several plates of pasta with bread and butter, and still be looking for dessert. Before surgery I had been required to go to a few classes, so logically I knew this was coming. Yet at that moment, I couldn't believe my flipping eyeballs. It was like I heard what they were saying in those pre-op classes, but now that I saw it right in front of me, I got it. Another Oprah "a-ha, light bulb moment" had just presented itself. I remember thinking "Ooooooh—that's what they meant by a 2 ounce meal." Holy crappits! What on earth had I gotten myself into? An immediate inner panic button went off. Right that second I realized that there was no turning back. It was like I had jumped off a cliff, not knowing whether or not my parachute was going to open.

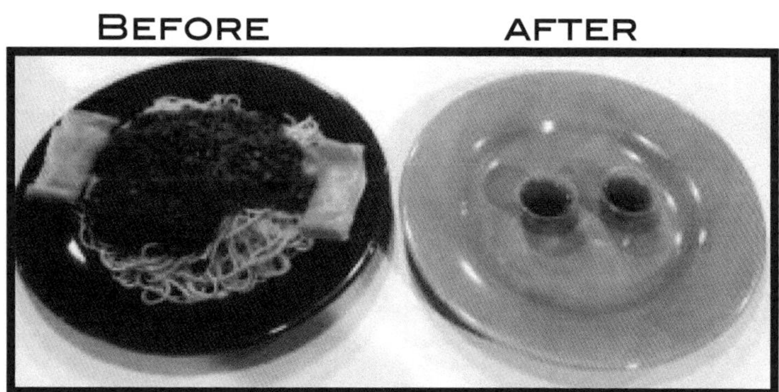

It's very hard to go hog-wild on chicken broth. Just saying.

No longer permitted to eat myself silly, now there was a list of foods I had to avoid. Let me translate "Avoid"...that's code for STAY THE HECK AWAY FROM! The pre-op information I had put on the back burner I was now forced to face head-on. Here are just a few of the things I was not allowed to consume: alcohol, carbonated anything, gum, peanut butter, bacon, nuts, greasy/fried foods, concentrated sweets, simple carbs (white bread, pasta, rice). Basically everything I lived on as 300-pound me.

avoid – to stay (the heck) away from or stop oneself from doing (something)

I was a baby all over again, using tiny spoons and drinking out of sippy cups. What a trip! The tiny spoons are used to remind you not to take giant bites. You have to go slow, eating very itty bitty spoonfuls. In the beginning it took me 30 minutes just to get that little bit of chicken broth and juice down the hatch. You can't drink out of a straw because slurping isn't allowed. The sippy cups are used to control the flow of fluid going in. You can't "chug" down a beverage in a sippy cup, and tiny spoons make it hard to scarf. And guess what? If you scarf, you will barf. Eating too fast, or eating the wrong foods can make you vomit and cause severe abdominal pain and cramping.

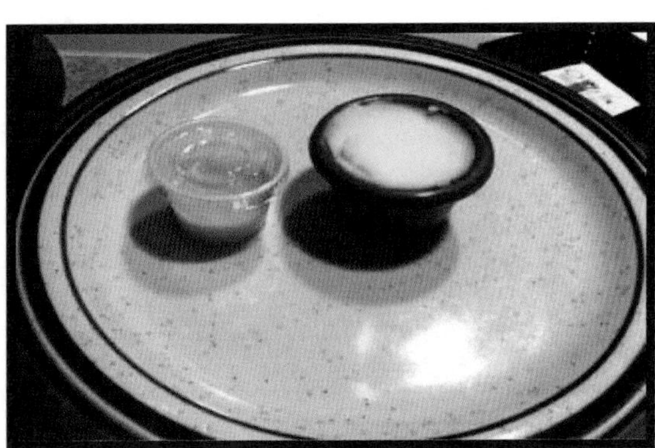

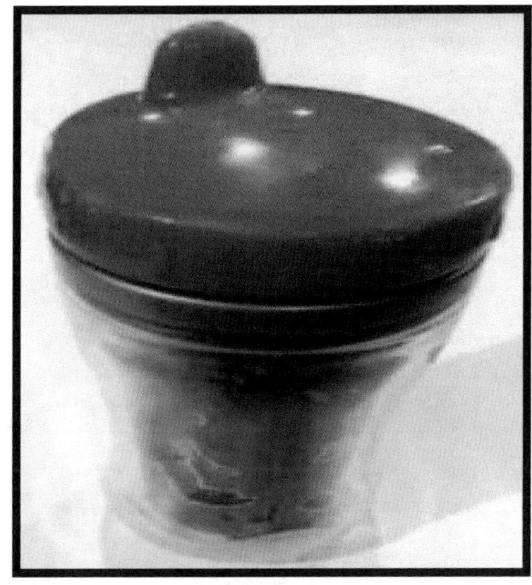

Three years since my surgery, I can eat pretty much like anyone else (that eats healthy), only smaller portions. To help with portion control, I never use anything bigger than a salad plate, and I eat about every two to three hours during the day. My pouch is now about 5 ounces, as they stretch a bit over time, which is expected.

Anyway, high protein foods are my fave. I absolutely love Greek yogurt, but it isn't for everyone. It is thicker in consistency (kind of like sour cream-thick), and pretty much you love it or hate it. If you are in the hate-it category, just grab another one that you do like. Yogurt is good for you, assuming you can tolerate lactose. Bariatric surgery changes things, and sometimes people can no longer tolerate milk. This can make meeting nutritional requirements hella-difficult. I am lucky; Milk and I are good buds. I go for the Greek yogurt because it's packed with protein. I eat it with a handful of nuts or granola. But let's be clear on the " handful situation". If your hand is huge you might be in trouble. Nuts are good, but they pack a fat gram punch. Keep it real, like one or two ('ish) ounces of nuts with a yogurt. It's a snack, not a meal, sister.

I'm all about squirrel snacks. That's my nickname for things like nuts, baked chips, granola (no added sugar), and pretty much anything that's whole grain and crunchy. I keep small portions of them with me. I absolutely stay away from regular chips or buttery crackers, which are what I would have eaten before, and before is no freaking more!

As far as carbs go, I didn't touch pasta, rice, bread, or potatoes for at least six months or so after surgery. This was not entirely by virtue I assure you, but merely by circumstance. Partially because I had no interest in them – which is stand-alone kruh-mazing (I used to survive on pasta). And, partially because they are just too hard to eat when you have a 2 ounce stomach. Bulky carbs don't stay down very well at first. Since my pouch is now 4-5 ounces, I can eat them in small quantities. Fortunately very small. If I overdo it, it feels like I swallowed a shoe, and it's horribly uncomfortable to the point it can make me throw up. I refuse to go the bariatric bulimic route. Scary thing is, I would bet my iPhone there are many bariatric patients making themselves puke because they overate the wrong foods and they don't want to regain their weight. Talk about deadly.

In the beginning, eating out was crazy-hard and more than just a teensy bit awkward. Portions are way out of whack for pretty much anyone at restaurants these days, but especially for the bariatric patient. I had to take my 1 ounce cups with me and measure out my food. No joke. Now I can pretty much go anywhere and find something to eat. I don't take 1 ounce cups with me anymore, but I don't get cocky either. I purposely do not go to places that serve unhealthy food, especially in gigantic portions. You have to set some boundaries for yourself as they pertain to food (duh). Mine include avoiding any all-you-can-eat situation and/or greasy, fast food. I used to live on it. Most fast food should be called "fat food." Anything dipped in grease and fried is clearly not good for you. If you look at most of the combos available at all of the major fast food chains it's always the same…a fried, greasy protein, fried or greasy carbs, and a soft drink. REALLY?! When did we all decide that was nutritious? Convenient and cheap maybe, nutritious NO! I would just grab and go, and continue to grow (I read a lot of Dr. Seuss as a kid, I can't help but rhyme). I could easily order 1000+ calories in one drive-thru run. Scary-true.

After surgery, I became aware of a huge trigger for me. The smells of food made me want to eat something! That's pretty normal actually, but now that I was a bariatric patient, things were different. I couldn't just go chowing down every time I caught a whiff of food that smelled good. I caught myself wanting to eat even though I had already eaten what I was supposed to and knew logically I was not hungry. How scary is that? I'm sure that reflex was there all along, but now I took notice because for the first time ever, I couldn't act on it with a tiny stomach.

A few weeks after surgery, I went to a state fair (which is like a scratch-and-sniff palooza for good food smells). I took one bite out of some type of scrumdidily-umptious meat sandwich, chewed it for a few seconds and had to spit it out. I had no business trying to eat it, and I knew it, but I attempted it anyway. NG. Anyhoo, I'm pretty sure they can (and will) deep fry anything at a state fair, so I'm not a fan of eating at them as a general rule. Last year I didn't go, but I heard there were things like deep fried Pepsi and even deep fried butter. REALLY?!!! Is that necessary? How do you freaking deep fry a Pepsi anyway? Some hillbilly out in the sticks has way too much time on their hands! Anyway, after my bariatric surgery, I became very aware of the connection between good food smells, and how they can trigger hunger for me. It may sound crazy, but when I can help it, I don't hang out where the food smells good. There are times this is unavoidable. When the unavoidable happens, I keep it real by point-blank asking myself if I am really hungry or if I am "fake hungry?" You know, eating because it smells good or, heck, just because I can reach it. Anyway, thank God I'm not Italian, or Chinese, or Mexican, or Peruvian because those folks invented making food smell good. Maybe I should get some nose plugs?

I've also taken bites of pizza and chips and done the same thing with the chew it, taste it, and spit it out business. NG. Thankfully, I got it out of my system, and now stay away from foods that can trigger cravings. If I hadn't, I know I would have returned to eating like I used to, and now that I've had bariatric surgery, that's not an option I want to explore. It's stuff like that that scares me. Dealing with food for me is so in my head. Maybe someday there will be a brain surgery that can just fix all of the psychological B.S. that goes along with eating.

While I am sure I could rationalize something to be marginally okay to eat at any fast food joint, I purposely stay away from all but a few of them. In fact, the instructions from my bariatric surgeon's office say, and I quote, "the wheels of your car should not touch a drive-thru for at least one year after surgery." I interpret that quote to mean...no drive-thrus EVER! I mean seriously, why reintroduce that whole scene? Has the food become that much better for you because they threw in a whole grain bun, apple slices, or added a salad packed with preservatives? Yeah...not so much. Another consideration is that even though there are some better choices available these days, would I actually make them once the smell of French fries wafted up my nose?

Today, I go places I can get lean protein and a salad that doesn't have a shelf life. I steer clear of pasta, bread, rice—you know the filler carbs—the ones that fatten me up. Bariatric surgery taught me how to eat right. I go for protein first, then whole grains and veggies. I would pick grilled chicken over a plate of pasta any day. A typical meal for me is about ¼ of a regular size entrée. The rest I take to go, or toss. It's very hard for me (and the clean-my-plate mentality) to throw food out, but it's even harder to hang on to it and contemplate eating it all day because it's "there" rather than because I am actually hungry. Way easier to toss it and kick "fake hungry" to the curb. I'm pretty sure overeating just because something is "there" wasn't the intention behind being conscientious with leftovers. Just saying.

When I said I never go to drive-thrus/fast food joints...I mean mostly never. My first stop every day is Mickey D's for a large coffee (or two), but that's it boss. No breakfast sandwich with a hash brown chaser these days. If I'm short on time and need to grab something on the fly, I go to places like Subway (You go Jared!). I might eat a ¼ to a ½ of a six inch sub with chicken breast and veggies, but that's the only sandwich I will order there. The processed meats anywhere might as well get in the state fair deep-fry line-up. They suck for your body! You can just taste the triglycerides. (BTW, a foot-long sandwich is ONE FOOT LONG). That's a lot of sandwich sister. Just saying. My all-time fave place to get something quick is Qdoba. I am not looking for any endorsements, I swear, but ask anyone who knows me – I bring it nearly every day for lunch. I go for beans, grilled chicken, lettuce, cheese, a dollop of sour cream, salsa, and a handful of chips. (*Remember the "handful situation" we talked about earlier). Since places like this are missing some things I like, I add some more stuff. I have a wonderful little trick I use every day. I call it "saladizing" – you can basically do it to any lunch or dinner meal. I take lettuce, Napa cabbage, spinach, cilantro, carrots, tomatoes and anything else I feel like, and chop it up and put it on top of my meal portion. For instance, I take 1/4 of Subway sandwich, or 1/5 of a Qdoba burrito, and saladize it up. Doing this allows me to eat smaller entree portions and add more veggies to my day. I use salsa as a dressing, or oil and vinegar, and it makes every meal salady. Yeah, that's right, I said…sal-add-ee. Give it a whirl! Instead of eating the entire burrito, cut it in fourths or a halves (whatever is right for you) and saladize it. You will be amazed how well this works for anyone, bariatric patient or not, plus you've just increased your veggie intake.

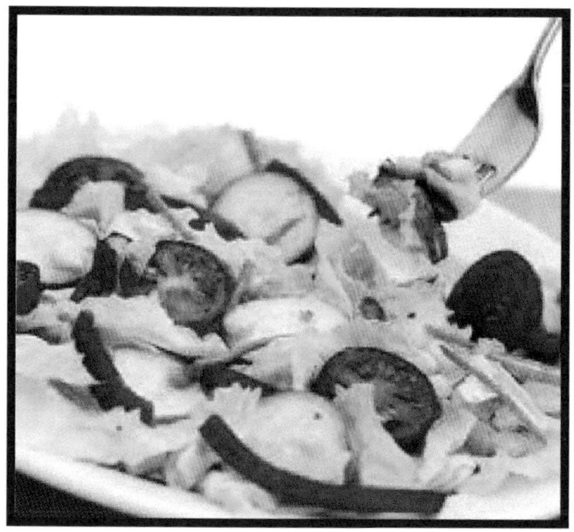

I combine saladizing with another lifestyle change that has had a huge impact for me. I don't go for the second carb serving we've all been asked to buy into. I don't need bread from a sandwich and then chips on top of that (not even baked ones). Really…all those carbs? If I eat slow over a ½ hour like I am supposed to, I will be full and not need the extra filler carbs. Besides, that is exactly how I used to roll with food…wolfing down tons of extra filler carbs. Oh, what's that? You need a refresher on what it means to actually sit down and eat for more than five seconds? If you're accustomed to scarfing down a few bites while skedaddling to the bathroom because you've had to pee for over an hour, then you need a refresher sister. We call it "multi-tasking". I call it running our hiney's off. O.K. skedaddler, go pee already (I'll wait for you).

WHEN ALL ELSE FAILS...GO PEE

—ROBANNE ROBIN

If you are a people-pleasing, "take one for the team" kinda gal (like myself), you need a reminder on a few things. How about a little sticky note quote? (Sure, why not).

#1 - Whatever it is you were doing can likely survive without you for 30 minutes. Seriously.

#2 - If not, call for reinforcements (unless of course you are launching a space shuttle or curing cancer or something, and the other guy that works with you has already gone on break).

#3 - Whenever possible, take a minute (or thirty) to walk away from the madness. Grab a breath of fresh air and some quiet. Take a few deep breaths and chew your food deliberately, preferably while sitting on your buns.

Before you go having a conniption fit, I already know what you are getting squwenchy about. How do you tell a toddler "Gone to lunch, back in 30 minutes?" Well, you don't. Nor would you leave any situation without someone covering you. That's the point. Get a wingman. Call for back-up. ASK FOR HELP. You may suck at that (like I did). But honestly, running yourself into the ground without taking a break doesn't do anyone a damn bit of good. If you need help finding a wingman, I've got you covered. Keep reading…I'll explain later, (but don't blink because you'll miss it).

I go everywhere prepared, EVERYWHERE. This is one of the hardest lifestyle changes I had to learn. It too, has had an enormous payoff. I pack a cooler for the car when I'm out and about for the day, even if I am just running to Target. Come on, girls...we all know a quick trip can easily turn into an expedition in a heartbeat. It's really no biggie,… just takes about an extra five minutes of planning before I hit the road. Take the whopping five minutes...you deserve it...your body deserves it. For example, I put one of the sugar-free teas I love, a can of diet soda, a water bottle, maybe a protein shake, a yogurt, sometimes some chicken and cheese slices. I may use none of it, some of it, or all of it depending on how long I am out. The point is I am prepared, and I don't let myself turn into Starvin' Marvin ready to go vulture on something. And just in case someone is walking around Target with French fry air freshener and the smell makes me hungry, I'll make it. I don't care what anyone thinks of my cooler – and be ready, people will say something. That's when I remind myself that if I put the same amount of effort into my wellbeing as I did into my food addiction, then I might have a chance. This kind of reality helps me dismiss outside influence. I know what I need to do, and I do it. Plain and simple. I dare to prepare when I'm out there (I love a rhyme). Best of all, now that I do it every day, it's cinchy.

I ALWAYS keep non-perishable dry snacks with me. I keep packets of instant (no sugar added) oatmeal, granola, nuts and baked chips in my trunk, gym bag, or my locker at work. That way, I always have good choices available to me. One of the best lifestyle changes I have made is to pack my lunch the night before! I don't care how tired I am. I do it. We both know how mornings can blow up when dealing with kids and many times you're just too tired to deal with packing your own lunch. Not to mention, if you are like me, pretty much nothing makes a tremendous amount of sense until I've had at least one cup o' Joe. Trying to pack a healthy lunch in a fog, in a rush, or even worse, in a foggy rush can be dicey.

By not preparing myself with healthy, available choices, I am actually setting myself up to excuse old behavior. I won't and don't allow myself to do that. It is up to me to set myself up for success by making healthy choices available to me. I think one of the things obese people fear is not having enough food and being hungry (at least I do). I think I still have that fear, and I don't know that "regular skinnies" get what I am talking about. That's o.k. I know it is real for me. Having control of fueling my body with healthy options empowers me to do the right thing and make healthy eating choices. The balance this brings to all areas of my life is kruh-mazing. BTW, I haven't had a French fry in over three years (no lie).

Part of my post-op bariatric diet plan includes not eating and drinking at the same time. In the beginning it was so I didn't get full too fast. Now, it's more so to protect me from myself. If I drink when I eat, I move food through my pouch quicker, therefore, getting hungry more often and eating more. I don't even want to go there, so I don't drink any beverages with my meals. (BTW, waitresses and waiters have no idea what to do with this). It throws them for a loop every time. Usually, they bring me water anyway, because it's just too hard not to apparently.

Anyhoo, somewhere along the way in life, I got it drilled into my head that variety with food was so important. While there is some truth to mixing it up so you don't get bored, I have found that routine and repetition work very well for me. Food is like a firecracker—dangerous to play with. If it works...go nuts and repeat meals that work for you as often as you want. This lifestyle change is awesome because for the most part, I don't have to rack my brain figuring out what I should eat. It's already done. For example, I eat instant plain oatmeal every morning for breakfast, and I freaking love it! It's easy-peasy, breezy, and cheap.

Before surgery, I was never a breakfast eater…or should I say a "regular" breakfast eater. Now put a plate of pancakes or biscuits and gravy in front of me back in the day, and all of a sudden, I could eat some breakfast. Heck, I could slather up those pancakes with butter, dump a ton of syrup on them, and then eat the biscuits and gravy too…no prob. Obviously, not the healthiest of choices. I was also good at eating a cholesterol-loaded breakfast sandwich along with a hash brown (or two)…but mind you…I would wash it all down with a "diet" soda. BTW, it is recommended not to drink any carbonated beverages for at least three to six months after surgery. Everyone's different, but it wasn't until nine months post-op that I could actually tolerate any carbonation. That's right, no bubbles, people. The fizzity-fizz-fizz irritated my stomach. I tried to take a sip of soda three months and four days after surgery (but who's counting), and it made me want to hurl. That was a trip – not drinking any soda or energy drinks, no carbonation PERIOD!

Now, I limit myself to one or two 12 ounce diet sodas a day. Prior to surgery, I used to drink a 12-pack of soda a day. I know it is just a can full of carbonated chemicals, but a girl's gotta have something. I also drink iced tea without sugar, and plenty of water. BTW, I don't drink alcohol and was advised not to for at least one year post-op. I didn't drink before the surgery, not even a drop, so it's no big whoop for me. From what I hear though, drinking alcohol with a 2-5 ounce stomach is the equivalent of giving a baby a drink. Zero to snookered in a few short sips. I don't plan on trying it. If you are a big drinker, that's going to be a deal-breaker for you, or at least it should be. Drunk baby - NG.

Today I pretty much do the exact same thing every day. I get my McDonalds coffee(s) for a buck a piece (God bless you Mickey D's), and I ask them for a small cup of hot water. They are going to hate me because they sell oatmeal...but oh well, I like mine better and I know what's in it (plus I am super picky). As I mentioned, I keep instant oatmeal packets in my glove box…and poof…there's breakfast! No matter how small the breakfast, I MUST eat it. My old lifestyle (usually) skipped breakfast, then gorged myself on a giant lunch, then a smattering of sugary snacks in between, followed later by a giant dinner, then dessert. Now mind you, the plain, heart-healthy, no sugar added oatmeal packet I use is only a mere 100 calories (hardly a sustainable breakfast). A few hours later, I do the Greek yogurt-squirrel snack situation which is another 300 ('ish) calories. I eat a small amount every several hours rather than pack it all down at once. A few hours later I will have a hardboiled egg (roughly 60 calories), and so on. I graze all day, eating smaller, snack-size meals and combine that way of eating with a whole bunch of exercise. BTW, I have no clue how many calories you should be eating. Get with someone who knows all that jazz and knows you, your health history, and your goals (preferably someone who has the initials M.D., or R.D. after their name). For the non-bariatric patients, please, for the love of God, don't follow some crazy, low-calorie deprivation diet. Kids cover your ears. It will backfire on you like seven cans of weight-gain whoop-ass.

The lifestyle changes I have implemented started with self awareness. It is dangerous territory for me to ask myself, "what do I want to eat…or what do I feel like eating?" – VERY BAD IDEA. For me that line of questioning allows cravings to take over, then the horse is out of the barn and food is flying the plane again. Mix cravings and emotions on high for 2 minutes, sprinkle in 1 cup of nerves and excitement, and a dash of uncertainty, and my friends you have emotional eating at its finest. (You can substitute any emotion if you are out of the ones I mentioned above). It becomes more about taste and not about nourishment and fueling the body. It turns into living to eat, rather than eating to live. I used any emotion good, bad, or indifferent as an excuse to chow down for far too long. Scooch over hog-wild, willy-nilly emotions. Those days are over Rover.

Right after surgery (especially), protein intake and hydration are essential. One of the most difficult things for me to manage was making sure I drank my protein shakes, and fluids every day, and that I took all of my liquid vitamins (that's right LIQUID vitamins...no pills larger than a baby aspirin allowed). I had to keep a schedule. At 7 a.m. drink this, at 9 a.m. take that, at 11 a.m. eat this, but don't drink a half an hour before or after a meal, and so on. This goes on all day long for months and months, and months. No joke. Saying this schedule is a challenge to keep up with is a monumental understatement. There are so many vitamins and nutritional supplements to manage for the bariatric patient specific to them and the type of surgery, so I am not going to even try to tackle that one. The point is, listen to your surgeon, follow the requirements, and meet with the dietician regularly. STAY ON TOP OF IT! All of this business requires a ginormous amount of "sticktoitiveness".

STICKTOITIVENESS (as defined by me):

STAYING ON IT LIKE WHITE ON RICE; HAVING A KUNG-FU GRIP ON YOUR GOAL

Time for another sticky note quote above the mirror (maybe we'll stick this one on the fridge):

> Dear Robanne:
>
> Just a reminder on a few things.
>
> #1 - You had freaking bariatric surgery.
>
> #2 - I don't really care if you don't feel like taking your liquid vitamins, or not drinking any beverages for 30 minutes before or after a meal, or having to actually sit down and take an entire half an hour to eat (no scarfing while skedaddling). Nor do I care if you want to drink your protein shake (which will take you all day in the beginning). Nor do I care if you want to exercise. Do it anyway.
>
> #3 - Just in case you are fickle (lazy) about doing anything in #2, please refer back to #1...You had freaking bariatric surgery! Good talk.
>
> Love,
>
> Your body

-WHEN IN DOUBT, I ASK MYSELF

"WHAT WOULD 300-POUND ME DO?" ONCE I HAVE THE ANSWER,

I RUN LIKE THE DICKENS IN THE OTHER DIRECTION-

Bariatric patients are prone to Protein Calorie Malnutrition (PCM) which can cause hair loss, muscle loss, slower healing time, and lack of energy. For the first 12 months after surgery, I was required to take in 75-90 grams of protein A DAY people. That's equivalent to having a baby eat about three hamburger patties daily. That's not going to happen without protein powder. Now, over three years since surgery, I can eat enough regular food to sustain me. I continue to drink protein shakes two to three times a week to help continue to build muscle as well as replenish the insane amount of calories I burn at the gym. I emphasize, I am intense (insane if you wish) when it comes to working out these days. I'll happily own that one. Now, a typical workout for me burns 750-1000+ calories (I've come a long way from the obese woman who could barely walk up the stairs without breaking a sweat). We'll talk exercise here in a minute, but it's hard for me to mention protein without touching on exercise and muscles. Anyway, I digress (again)...back to protein. It's just good fuel for the bod. It makes me feel amazing, full of energy, and here's the best of one of all, I'M NOT AS HUNGRY. It has something to do with protein taking longer to digest than carbs, so you have more energy and not constantly craving more carbs ...yada...yada...yada (please consult with those who are trained professionals on this one). BTW, just because someone is "certified" does not make them good. For example, if you meet with a dietician or fitness instructor who weighs 300 pounds…there's your first clue to skedaddle.

The breakthrough for me has been to learn how to eat and nourish my body for the first time in my life. In my late 30's, I finally started to fuel my body wisely. It's just like gassing up a car. If you don't fill up, it won't run (for long). My body is no different, it can't operate on fumes, or with a bunch of junk in the trunk. While I remain very aware of the foods to avoid, I make it a point to focus on the list of foods I can have (which is much longer). By doing this, I take the whole "I can't have it sob story" right out of the picture. And even though I am A-O.K. with repeating what I'm eating, I challenge myself to try new things now and again. But, as a general rule, I keep food as simple as I can and I don't fall in love with it. It's just freaking food! We don't have to hunt and gather anymore, there's a grocery store on every corner, so it's not necessary to eat everything in sight. Food is fuel to power my body, that's it. For me, protein = GOOD. Simple carbs and refined sugar = VERY BAD. As important as nourishing my body is, I had to take it a step further and do the unthinkable for 300-pound me. Holy crappits and f-bombs, I had to freaking exercise!

-ASK YOUR DOCTOR IF GETTING OFF YOUR BUTT IS RIGHT FOR YOU-

(I love this one, so you will see it again)

9

God, the Radio and Exercise

They told me I would have to exercise after the surgery…"30 minutes of walking EVERYDAY." Sounds doable, right? Would you believe that after the surgery I was ready to renege? At first I thought, nanny-nanny boo-boo, I got my surgery so screw you! The weight's going to come off anyway, right? Then my old thinking piped up… "I don't feel like exercising." Honestly, for the first month or so after the surgery I did the bare minimum in the exercise department. I walked a little and rode my bike slowly around the neighborhood a little. By "a little", I mean maybe two or three times a week for (maybe) 15 minutes tops, never breaking a sweat (not exactly what I had agreed to before surgery). I knew I should be doing more, but at the same time the weight was starting to drop off, so I was like…"whatevs, I'm cool." I began rationalizing..."the exercise part just won't be my strong suit". Loosely translated, "I was never planning on changing my lifestyle anyway". Besides, I was very compliant with the food rules and pretty much followed all of that to the T (except for random bites of meat sandwiches at state fairs). I figured I had some leeway, right? WRONG. I was so wrong, but I didn't know it yet. SCREW YOU almost became SCREW ME.

Right after surgery, I was barely hungry. Although only temporary, it was a freakishly kruh-mazing experience for a girl who's been hungry her whole life. I was only able to eat a very tiny bit at first. Everyone is different, but it took months and months for me to even care about food. Here's the weirdest part, for six to nine months, I did not crave any sugar or carbs - I'm talking NADA ENCHILADA! I swear they must have operated on my brain. I remember Halloween came and went and I didn't touch even one piece of candy. Here's the kruh-mazing part—I didn't even want to! Pump the breaks and listen up sisters. This pseudo-immunity did not last forever. Those days came to a screeching halt. ERRRRRRRRRRCK!

I started to want carbs and sugar again. It was like…POOF! They were back on my radar screen (sneaky bastards), although not nearly in the way they were before. Heck, prior to bariatric surgery, I could whack an entire store-bought cake, or a pint of ice cream (1000 calories in one shot) with absolutely no problem. The desire that returned was not enormous like that, but I could eat sugar and carbs again, and it scared the ba-jeezus out of me. What if I am able to just keep eating more and more…and then one day, I am eating an entire sheet cake again? I know what I am capable of and it makes me cringe. I am now hungrier, and can eat far more than before. No wonder bariatric patients re-gain their weight! Old habits die hard, old thinking dies even harder. People eat the foods they should stay the heck away from, their tires are touching the drive-thrus, their stomach stretches back out, they don't exercise, therefore there is no lifestyle change, and they regain the weight. That's the Cliff Notes explanation. Try Google-ing "bariatric non-compliance" for the long version, or better yet, go talk to a bariatric surgeon. Here's the BIG POINT (again): Just because you surgically alter the size of someone's stomach, it does not alter the super-sized thinking that got them out of shape in the first place. It doesn't change old habits and behaviors. You can (and will) eat more and more as time goes on, and if you don't exercise, and sugar and carbs show back up on the radar screen then... BAM! YOU ARE HOSED! If I had not made the lifestyle changes in the first six to nine months, I would not be where I am at today. Making the leap from the couch to the treadmill was crazy-hard, and I almost didn't do it, but that was all about to change.

A little over three months out from surgery I was once again having the mental debate in my head… "go to the gym Robanne…nah, but I don't want to…but you should go…but I don't feel like it…but what about that half an hour-a-day business you had agreed to?…I really should go…but I really DON'T want to." I am not sure what possessed me to get my butt up off the couch, get in the car and head out to the gym, but I did. Maybe it was one of those sticky notes I put up? Anyway, that one decision at about three o'clock in the afternoon on a chilly November day changed the course of my life as a bariatric patient. My success hinged upon it, and I had no idea at that moment just how important taking the action to do something I did not want to do would ultimately be. I am convinced that if I had not budged and succumbed to the (all-day) nap I wanted to take, I would not be where I am today. I would have merely been marking time, only to be setting myself up for failure and a return to 300-pound me.

Anyway, it's November and a bit nippy out – another reason for my head to win the battle for me not to go to the gym. I get in the car anyway, my head still trying to talk me out of going to get my agreed upon half hour of exercise. Like that mattered now. I got what I wanted, so we're done, right? I turn on the radio randomly, as I normally listen to CD's. Yeah, I said CD's. It means "compact disc" for those of you who have forgotten. I hadn't joined the iPhone mafia yet, and even if I had, my '95 Chrysler Cirrus didn't roll with an MP3 player. So anyhoo, on the radio is this guy who was a former Biggest Loser winner or contestant or something (I can't remember). He starts talking about how he has lost all his weight and how essential it was for him to make lifestyle changes in order to keep it off...yada, yada, yada. Then it hit me…he's freaking right! If I don't change my old behaviors and change my lifestyle…then WTH was the surgery for? You would think one might have figured that out *before* undergoing bariatric surgery, but in my case, not so much. Anyway, who cares because at that moment, (which is really all that matters) I GOT IT. In my car of all places, the message I most needed to hear came to me over the radio. It was EXACTLY what I needed to hear, EXACTLY when I needed to hear it. That radio dude was talking DIRECTLY TO ME and although I am not a super religious girl, I have to believe that moment and that message were divinely orchestrated for me to hear. I can hardly believe that in the 2.3 miles from my house to the YMCA, that was the message I was blessed to hear, and that I was paying attention and ready to hear it (that helps). During that five minute window of time, this pivotal moment happened. It was my moment of clarity…that holy crappits, "Oprah aha moment," so to speak (I have a lot of those, thank goodness).

-OLD HABITS DIE HARD

OLD THINKING DIES EVEN HARDER-

It was then that it dawned on me that there are so many people that aren't as fortunate as I am. They are far too sick and weak to even contemplate taking on my challenge. In that moment, I realized – I'm fat, I'm not dead. If my thinking were a gear shift, I literally put it into reverse and did a 180. Ironically, after taking the action to go to the gym (which I totally did not want to do), I began to realize that I *get* the opportunity to go work out. I am relatively healthy enough to be able to do it. What a quality problem it is to have to fit exercise into my busy life, full of blessings. What a nice way to see things. Try it. Time for another sticky note quote. This one we will put on the couch:

Dear Robanne,

#1- Couches are for sitting intermittently. They are not for taking all-day naps in front of the TV when you haven't gone to the gym (or even if you have).
#2 - Get off the couch.
#3 - Don't make me come over there.

Good Talk. Love,

Your Body

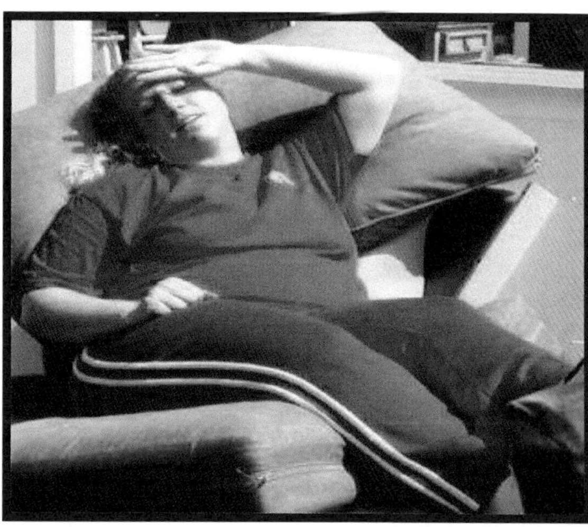

You know things are meant to be when you are writing about getting off the couch and you actually stumble across a photo of your 300-pound-self sprawled out on one.

So I roll up to the Y that has made all of the difference in my transformation. I don't think I could have survived my own thoughts in a hoity-toity, fancy pants, fu-fu gym. Not that the Y isn't nice, but I have found it to be way more down-to-earth and fam-friendly. And, while every gym has its posse of beach Barbies in their 20's, the one's at the Y have at least given birth. I'm just going to say it. It's harder than heck for an obese person to walk into to a gym. It's a victory just to make it through the front door, let alone try and survive their own head and the self-defeating thinking that is working against them even before they pulled into the parking lot.

The folks at the Y cheered me on and helped my family too. They have child care included in the membership (there goes that excuse). BTW, a fitness center with childcare makes an excellent wingman. I was able to drop off the little trolls for up to two hours so I could exercise. Priceless! Please understand, I mean "trolls" with love. That expression is kind of like "rug-rats," but with crazier Don King hair.

Now I'm all hopped up on the..."Y-M-C-A...I'm talking 'bout the Y-M-C-A." It's there I learned to replace the "G" word, you know, "gym." At the Y they call it the "wellness center." What a beautiful thing to call it! After all, it's about getting well…not getting "gymned." I became determined not to be "that guy" that goes through all of this, only to gain all of the weight back and then some. There are many of "those guys" out there. In fact many bariatric patients re-gain all their weight. I bet you will find the odds are not forever in your favor in terms of achieving long-term success after bariatric surgery, (or any method of weight loss) if you don't rock the lifestyle changes. Speaking of which, I recently read somewhere that you are not considered "successful" unless you have kept your weight off for at least five years. Technically, I am still two years shy of being a success. Okey dokey. I'll write another book in two years when I hit the five-year mark (promise). So keep in mind as you read my story, I'm still "iffy."

I am no expert and probably know enough to be dangerous on any given day, but what I can tell you is what I have experienced and what I have seen. Sorry to burst your bariatric bubble, but there is no way someone can have this surgery and ride off happily into the healthy lifestyle sunset without doing the work to get there (and stay there). If you are truly considering bariatric surgery, you need to know what you are up against. I'm not going to Splenda-coat it for you...YOU'RE UP AGAINST A LOT. But don't let me discourage you. After all, I am your average, everyday blend of ignorance and courage, and I have done just fine.

Honestly, I can't say I totally disagree with this five-year success business. Workout rooms at many bariatric centers are lights out, dead empty every time I'm there. Better yet, just go to one of the bariatric support group meetings and you'll see what I'm talking about. The rate of recidivism is astounding. No…it's more than astounding…it scares the heck out of me. I don't know what the stats are off-hand of bariatric patients that regain all of their weight, but check into it, or ask a bariatric surgeon. Remember, this book is a diary of my own experience and not a stats book (let someone else more qualified write that one).

Anyway, I've gone to some bariatric support group meetings. A lot of valuable (I'm talking priceless) information can be obtained by what you see right before your very eyes—so pay attention when you're out there. Besides, everyone is an example, good or bad. I respect and thank those who are willing to share what they've done right or wrong. It's up to me to set the actions in motion that I need to take, and be the example I want to be. At the last meeting I went to, I took a seat and looked around. Holy mother of @#! Most everyone in the room who had previously had bariatric surgery had plumped right back up. I was like this freakish anomaly. Some of them were now considering a revision which is basically a do-over of their bariatric surgery. A revision! REALLY? I am not sure where this falls on the OMG-this-is-dangerous scale, but it's up there. Ask any bariatric surgeon worth their weight in Krugerrands, and if they're honest, you'll get an earful. Some docs won't even do revisions because they are crazy-dangerous, (as if the original bariatric surgery wasn't enough of a risk).

Listen, I'm on your side, I really am. But, (there's always a but), if you are "that guy" that's had bariatric surgery and been non-compliant, then you seriously need to change what the heck you are doing. BTW, "non-compliant" is code for: you had bariatric surgery and didn't change a damn thing. Ask yourself how that's working for you? Get a pen, write this down and put it on your bathroom mirror, your fridge and your couch (and anywhere else you'll see it). For the umpteenth time, this surgery DOES NOT change your obese thinking. If you change nothing, guess what? YOU CHANGE NOTHING. Remember the definition of insanity here people. Even worse, remember that beneath insanity lies the trap door of indifference. You must change EVERYTHING.

Bottom line (again): exercise and diet must go together. Now, wait a minute. I'm going to stop right there and say this: the word diet has the word "die" in it. I don't hate much, but I hate that flipping word. Diets alone don't work or else I wouldn't be writing this book. Let's just call it "eating and nourishing" your body, with the caveat that if the word "diet" creeps its way back in, you know what I'm saying. Ok, I feel better now. Where were we? Oh yeah…the bottom line is exercise and nourishment must go together. They're like this (fingers crossed). You can't do just one…you need BOTH to equal a lifestyle change (and don't get me wrong, I'm sure you need some other stuff too). We'll talk about "other stuff" in a bit.

The fact that I have lost half of my body weight is ridiculously kruh-mazing! Is that even possible? Apparently, it is. I call it the Holy Snikeys Factor (or HSF for you texters). Feel free to use holy crap or holy moly if holy snikeys doesn't sink your Cheerios. I talked with my surgeon not only about how much weight I have lost, but also the unexpected level of fitness I have achieved. She said to me, "I wish you would go to a bariatric support group meeting and tell everyone how important it is to exercise." I thought back to the last meeting I had gone to, and another Oprah a-ha, light bulb moment occurred which got me thinking (and writing). I have something to share that would benefit others! Heck, if I can spare anyone from voluntarily going head-first into a ditch (like I almost did), then I'm all about it.

Okay, so let's review? Diets (ugh…that word again), it's like you can't get away from it. Anyway, those freaking things alone don't work…agreed. Exercise is MANDATORY (as in NOT OPTIONAL)…check. Wait a minute…let's stop there. I didn't exactly embrace the exercise component from day one…not even from day 61. So how did I get where I am now? Well, after the radio revelation I mentioned, I decided to commit to the half hour a day of cardio that I said I would do all along. Wasn't that big of me, to comply with the rules I had agreed to prior to having the surgery? I began walking on the treadmill at a 4.0 clip. I would do about a mile and a half in 30 minutes, then I got a little faster and was able to do 2 miles in 30 minutes. After several months of this, all along still dropping about 15-20 ('ish) pounds a month from the bariatric surgery, I was really feeling good.

I began to think…what if I jogged a teensy bit? Couldn't hurt right? After all, no matter how slow I go, I am still lapping the guy on the couch, right? RIGHT! Anyway, I was pretty slow, starting off at 5.0-5.4, which is roughly an 11-12 minute mile. I was kind of like a turtle, slow and steady. Before I knew it, I was knocking down 3 miles in 30 minutes (impressive for former 300-pound me). Then one night at the gym, this gal was running next to me - I mean hauling A sisters. At the risk of being a lookie loo, I nonchalantly glanced over and saw her speed of 7.0 (equivalent to an 8 ½ minute mile), and I thought "that will never happen for me." There were many moments like that. Moments where my own inner voice was by far my worst enemy, tearing me down, telling me I would not make it. If you have that voice, (and you know you do)…do yourself a favor as I did…and tell it to STHU or STFU (who am I to censor you?). I consciously make a decision on a regular basis not to get sucked into that negativity. I just won't let it take me down. I stop the thought by replacing it with a simple phrase we've all overused…YOU GO GIRL (YGG)! That's right…"you go Robanne," I would say to myself. "Way to not be 3-hundy sitting around (probably on the couch) eating yourself to death. Way to be at the Wellness Center working to make a positive change in your life!" I said it before, and I'll say it again (and probably again after that)...no matter how slow you go, you're still lapping the guy on the couch. Can I get an Amen, sisters?

Exercise tip numero to the uno...GET YOUR MUSIC ON! I LOVE my iPod/iPhone thingy (move over old school cd's, I have one now). It has the music I LOVE on it, and for my workout, that makes all the difference. Get your music on, friends. Go ahead…put a little boom in it! It helps, and if you're like me, you need all the help you can get! You might also need a 13-year-old to be your IT director so you can learn how to use the darn thing. One more tidbit, you might also need some therapy after you drop and shatter your smexy new iPhone. It's all fun and games until you take it out of the case.

Anyway, a few months after I began to jog, I started to add in weights (controlled resistance, actually no free weights at all). Controlled resistance is fancy for "the machines". I alternate legs one day and then arms the next. That breaks down to Monday, Wednesday, Friday on the arms, and Tues., Thurs. for legs. Weekends are a little random with work...besides, a girl needs a rest day here and there. I focus more on my arms because I LOVE the definition, and OMG, no one can flipping believe how ripped my arms are – I can hardly believe it!

I am not much of an early morning exerciser, never have been, (and if I can help it…never will be). Although on rare occasions, I do make a 5 a.m. cameo appearance (that's if I can't go workout when I'm actually awake). Anyway, what gives, you ask? Well, my entire life I thought I was doomed unless I worked out before the sun came up. Seriously. I always had this preconceived notion that you had to get up at the A-crack of dawn to be physically fit. But NO...NO you don't. <u>YOU</u> have to do it when <u>YOU</u> can do it, in a manner in which <u>YOU</u> can consistently do it. So if early mornings are your thing, then go nuts, chicken wing. But, it's okay if they are not. Honestly, I don't know which is harder...going to the gym at the A-crack of dawn before work, or schlepping in after a long day? So figure out which one sucks less for you, pick your fave, and do it! My experience with a successful fitness routine has been to do what I can do consistently. That's why I like the half-an-hour-a-day concept. It's not crazy. It's actually achievable and maintainable. Now, I regularly do much more than a half hour.

-NO MATTER HOW SLOW YOU GO, YOU'RE STILL LAPPING THE GUY ON THE COUCH-

(UNLESS THE COUCH IS ON AN AIRPLANE OR SOMETHING, IN WHICH CASE YOU ARE GETTING SMOKED).

I find it VERY helpful to commit to a group exercise class because it's easier to show up when I have to be accountable to others that are expecting me to show up! The treadmill doesn't really give a rat's-A if I show up or not. Here's an idea: go crazy and get to know some of the regulars in the gym. I mean like actually talk to them and get to know their names. While we as a society have some crazy-strong opposable thumbs, you've got to admit, that like our kids, we've lost the fine art of actually interacting with other humans we don't know (except for maybe a text or email). For years I didn't talk to anyone at the gym, I was so self-conscious it was ridonculous. Today I look at it differently. We are all in this exercise thing together, with a commonality that binds us. Heck if that's too deep, how about the commonality that we are all making an effort to get off the couch? That'll work. Plus it's nice to have someone to say "hi" to. Actually, at the end of my hip hop class, it's like a chickity-chat palooza! I have met the coolest people with all kinds of backgrounds and interests…professional dancers, nurses, fitness pros, stay at home mommy-worker bees, doctors, social workers, students, custodians, and this one really cool lady who is legally blind, but rocking a hip hop class with some serious hi-powered bifocals. YGG!

I usually workout somewhere between 9-11 a.m. or 4-6 p.m. because that is what works for my life (at the moment). We all know how life likes to go and effing change on us. So when that happens, I get a little squwenchy about having to re-arrange things, then I get over myself and make it happen. The key here is <u>what works</u>. If it doesn't work, it will not last. If you don't enjoy it, guess what, you won't do it. Now…when I say "enjoy" it, I don't mean you have to love it…you just don't have to hate it! One way I figure that part out is by trying something new every few months. I still do my regular workout, but I find it interesting to see what the read-out is on the love-it, hate-it, or kinda-like-it barometer when I step out of my comfy zone. I keep an open mind here. I mean, if I think about it, how the heck do I know what exercise I like? I was 300 pounds for like 10 years (not exactly tearing down the exercise path). If you are anything like me, what you kinda like, you may grow to love. You'd be surprised. That's how I fell into hip hop, yoga, and TRX training! I love kettle bells too (lie). Those damn things are medieval, but at least I tried it. What's important is that I let my fraidy-cat self step out of my comfy zone and dare to try something new. Super scary, but I am so glad I did it! As a result of trying new things, I have gone from someone who was never going to be a runner, to having the capability of running a 7:30 mile. The Jamaican's are safe from me, but that's no chump change.

But don't be a knucklehead. If you have bad knees – which I'm guessing you might if you've been toting around the weight of an extra person like I was for a decade – you have no business running right out of the gate (or maybe ever). I'm not trying to be the boss of you, but you know I'm right. So please for the love of God, don't go hauling off on some extreme boot camp, P-1-billion X, Cross Stitch, Plyo-Insane-in-the-membrane workout plan UNTIL you have gotten the green light to do so from your doctor. Pump the brakes grasshopper! If you are as far out of shape as I was, it will take a while for that light to turn green. Once you get the initial hi-sign from the doc, then get with a good personal trainer and set some realistic goals. I know everyone wants to be "fixed" in a one-hour session, but let's be real. You didn't get out of shape in an hour. Follow up regularly with your doc and trainer and advance appropriately. Is this chick for real? Personal trainer, in this economy? Now, I know that sounds all big-time having a trainer and all...but chillax before you get all squwenchy on me. I get that not everyone can afford a PT...well, guess what...me neither (kinda). I can't afford a fu-fu gym membership with a she-she personal trainer, but I can swing a family membership at the local Y which I have discovered has very reasonable PT rates with kruh-mazing trainers. BTW, I haven't crunched all the numbers, but I'm pretty sure a membership at the Y and a PT session once a week or so is a bazillion times cheaper than heart disease, diabetes, stroke...and I don't know...DEATH! It's certainly cheaper than the $20 ('ish) bucks I spent daily on drive-thrus and dessert runs. You do the math.

> **"Finding the right person(s) to help you set and achieve attainable goals is essential to your healthy lifestyle. You should always speak to your physician before starting any new exercise regimen."**
>
> **—Matthew G. Newmann, MS, ACSM-CPT, M.S. Kinesiology**

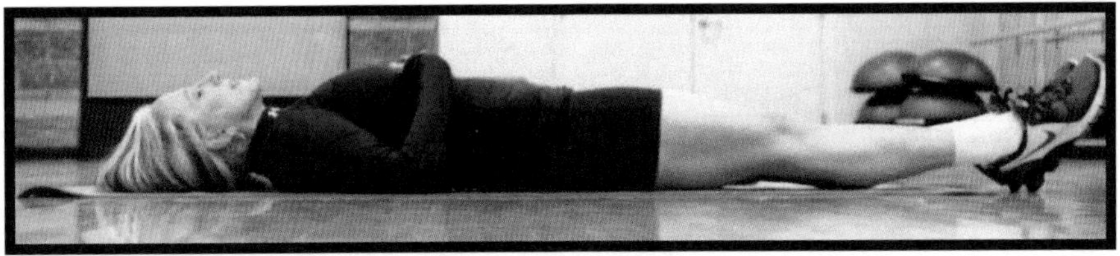

When it comes to exercise, eating right (or anything really)...

YOU DON'T HAVE TO LOVE IT...

YOU JUST DON'T HAVE TO HATE IT

THAT'S NOT SWEAT, IT'S LIQUID AWESOME

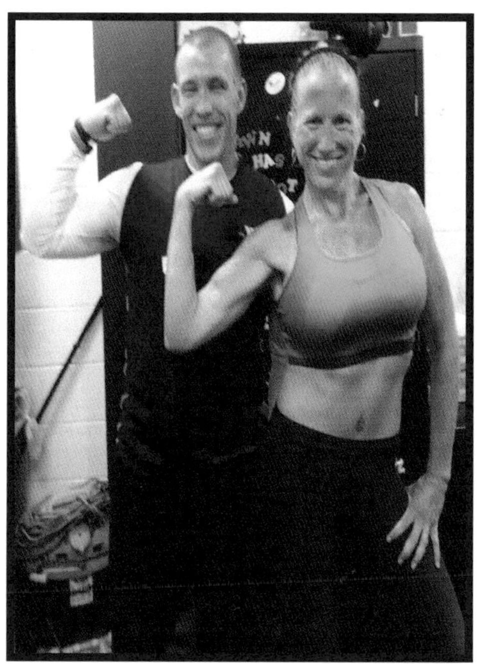

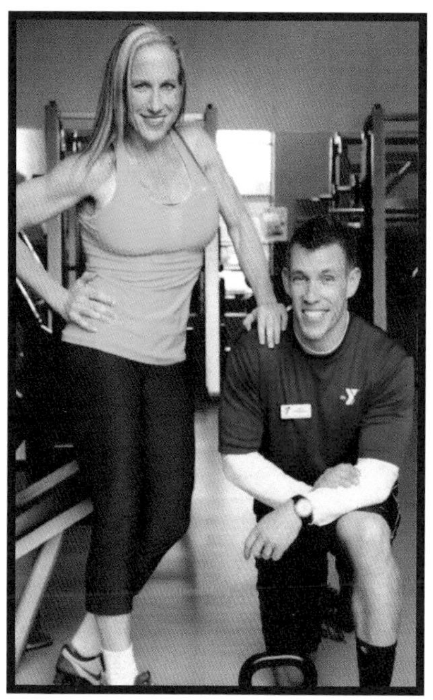

Photo with Matthew G. Newmann, A.C.S.M., C.P.T., M.S. Kinesiology
It would be much easier if I just put "rock star" after his name.

The photo on the left was taken on August 4, 2012 with my trainer Matt Newmann, exactly 3 years since my bariatric surgery. That is a very special day I will always honor with a photo and a big 'ol smile (& probably a hands on my hip, bicep flex pose for good measure).

Here it is again…

-ASK YOUR DOCTOR IF GETTING OFF YOUR BUTT IS RIGHT FOR YOU-

If you are anything like I was, you paid the gym membership fees, but never actually went to the gym. How many years did I do that for? Don't be that guy; go nuts and get into the gym! Let 'em scan your tag and show up on the radar screen! Show up for you. You deserve it! I remember one time it had been so long since I had actually, physically walked through the front doors that I was afraid they would be able to detect my hiatus when they scanned my card. "And making her annual appearance...we have Robanne Robin." Geez-Louise my head is my own biggest enemy! No one cares. Really. So no matter how long it has been...get over yourself and get your buns moving for at least 30 minutes a day, whether it is at the Y or walking in your neighborhood. If you have a pair of tennis shoes and you can walk, then you can do this. Break a good sweat. Once you've been able to maintain that consistently for a few months ('ish) start to add in the extras like weights, fancy classes, etc. (preferably under the specific direction of someone trained in these matters).

Like I said—don't be a knucklehead! I had to work my way up to advanced group exercise classes. Don't set yourself up for failure (you're probably as good at that as I am). Not to mention, you can hurt yourself. Advanced classes are no joke, and should not be attempted on a whim. I mean seriously, some of these classes have more accessories than my pre-teen daughters…sheesh! Bosu balls, bands, weights, benches, bars, kettle bells. That's too much in the beginning…be smart and work up to it. Once, they had to call an ambulance for a lady who was in over her head and passed out. So check yourself before you wreck yourself. It's about progression, not perfection. Start slow, baby steps. Pushing too hard doesn't equal instant results. It took about a year for me to even see a muscle. Then, sha-BAM! There they were...hello. Your timeline might be different. Be patient grasshopper. Keep at it, and remarkable things will happen. By "remarkable," I mean stuff that wouldn't be happening while napping on the couch.

Some classes are just not my thing, nor will they be yours (like the Zumba...too many salsa-ee jazz-hands and spirit fingers for this kid, but I have friends that won't shut up about it--and they shouldn't!). If you love it, you'll do it! For girlfriend here, the most important challenge is to try new things. Now I know I said I'm all about repetition when it comes to food, but exercise is different. I've never gone off track with exercise and gotten lost for a decade. Exercise is a much safer area for me to dabble around in. Go ahead. Stick a toe in the waters that lie just outside your comfy zone (crazy-scary I know, but if I can do it, so can you, sister). Go discover what you like. Keep the workouts interesting and fun along with physically challenging (within reason). It's so important to mix up your routine a little. No one can do the same workout everyday forever. They just can't. Number one, you risk boredom (which means you won't keep at it), and more importantly you risk injury (which speaks for itself). Either one of those can take you right out of the exercise game. Not a game I can afford to be out of. By mixing it up, you may just find something you love, that you never would have known you loved unless you tried it.

Recently, I tried turbo kick…AWESOME! I somewhat suck at it since I am new to it, but who cares? You get to air-punch your bippies off, so it's totally worth sucking. It's a choreographed class just like Hip Hop Hustle, which means it starts with a new routine every so many weeks, and it keeps repeating until the next new one starts. So, if you walk into one of those classes, and you are completely lost, you're kind of supposed to be. You'd be a freak of nature if you just walked in and nailed it. Give it a chance, go back at least a few times before you quit, or better yet, just keep at it and suck! You may pick it up like I did with Hip Hop Hustle. What a happy accident finding that class was for me! I literally stumbled upon it when I ventured into unknown territory. One day these gals were standing in the gym going on and on about how awesome this class they just took was. Curious George here was dying to know WTH they had discovered, so I asked them. Ever since, I have been officially hooked on Hip Hop Hustle! If you hit a hip hop class, check your minivan keys at the door sisters because (not that you need it), but you have my full permission to shake what your mama gave ya. You'll be glad you did! Minivan mom's love Hip Hop Hustle (MVM's ❤ HHH). I still don't own a minivan, but you get the point...drop the kids off, dust away the dry Cheerios on your (hopefully sassy) t-shirt and go for it! I have never had so much fun burning calories. Whether it's hip hop hustle or pickle ball, go find your fun sisters. It's out there! You think I'm joking with the pickle ball…nope it's really a sport.

I start yoga again soon (YAY)! Yoga is the counter-balance of all the extreme exercise I do. It stretches and aligns me, and talk about working out some kinks. Man. I am like a human bendy straw, it's nuts. For me yoga is so important because it's "stretchy" (that's a fun word). Say it again…"stretchy". It's a great way to improve strength and flexibility without pounding all of my joints into the ground, and talk about chillaxing. Anyway, now for a brief stretching lecture. While I am a stretching fool, many people rush that part, or let's be honest, don't do it at all. Don't skimp on the stretching, sisters! As my friend JoLynn would say, "Stretch yourself before you wreck yourself".

-STRETCH YOURSELF BEFORE YOU WRECK YOURSELF-

–JoLynn Wright

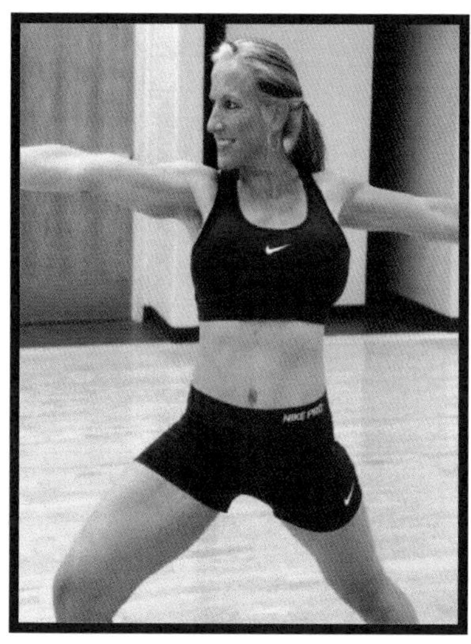

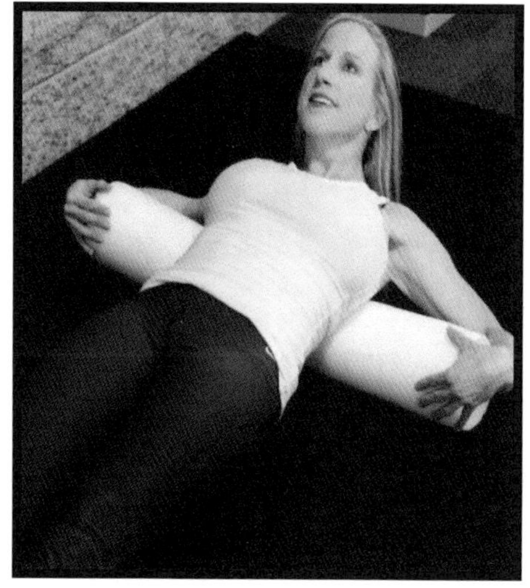

A note about group exercise instructors: They are not all created equally! Especially, when there is a sub, (and there will be one from time to time), you may not get the same workout. If you are me, you are there to work out and you mean business. There were several times when I just suffered through the hour, barely breaking a sweat. Then, it dawned on me… I don't have to be rude, but I certainly do not have to stay (duh). My workout time is precious and hard to come by at times (sound familiar?). I am going to get my money's worth during that hour, girlfriends. I have walked out of several classes when I know I just won't get the workout I need, and I hit the treadmill for an interval workout. I just don't play. I have come too far to pretend anymore, and I have a healthy fear of a return to Fatty McButterpants, USA. It's not a place I ever want to call home again.

Check this goal out...I want to teach a hip hop class. Me! Who on earth knew that underneath that 300-pound exterior was a hip hop maniac waiting to break free? I betcha it will happen. For several years I have been like a hip hop stalker and take almost every class at the Y. So who better to teach a class when I heard they needed a substitute instructor? I just knew yours truly should be the one! Feeling somewhat like when I was a teenager filling out my first job application at Weinerschnitzel (a job I did get by the way), I filled out the paper form and applied to be a fill-in hip hop instructor. And, SHAZAM! I got the "thanks for your interest" email, not even an interview. Actually I'm embellishing. I got no reply at all, and when I followed up on my application, that's when I got the "thanks, but no thanks" reply. You know what, I could let that get the old undies in a squwenchy bunch, or I could decide that I am supposed to focus my energies and efforts in other areas right now. Since you are reading this book, you guessed which one I chose. No hard feelings, the Y is awesome and I love them! Either way, I still got my hip hop certification, because I wanted it. Maybe one day they'll let me put it to use and give me my first hip hop instructor break (hint! hint!). The fact that I've migrated from someone who could barely take the class, to getting hip-hop certified and applying to teach it is totally kruh-mazing! YGG! (I cheer for myself now and again).

.

-MAKE TODAY RIDICULOUSLY AMAZING-

(EVEN IF "TODAY" IS A COMPLETE WASTE OF MAKEUP)

Things happen for a reason. I have to believe that. When what I thought I was supposed to get or what I wanted didn't happen, it's always been because I needed to be freed up to do what I didn't know was coming. I often simmer on that when I am feeling all of the glory and splendor of rejection life occasionally likes to serve up. Let me tell you, there's no shortage of rejection and disappointment out there. Just try and write a book and you'll see what I'm talking about. Even so, don't let anyone or anything discourage you. Besides, if you are like me, you're pretty good at discouraging yourself and you don't require any assistance.

I remind myself: YOU decide how smart you are. YOU decide how hard you are going to work. YOU are your own gatekeeper, no one else. For too much of my life I have let what others think and say determine my actions. This book may be nothing but a coaster when I am done (well, actually 1,000 coasters, but who's counting?). However, I will have done it and spared myself the years of wondering "what if I had?"

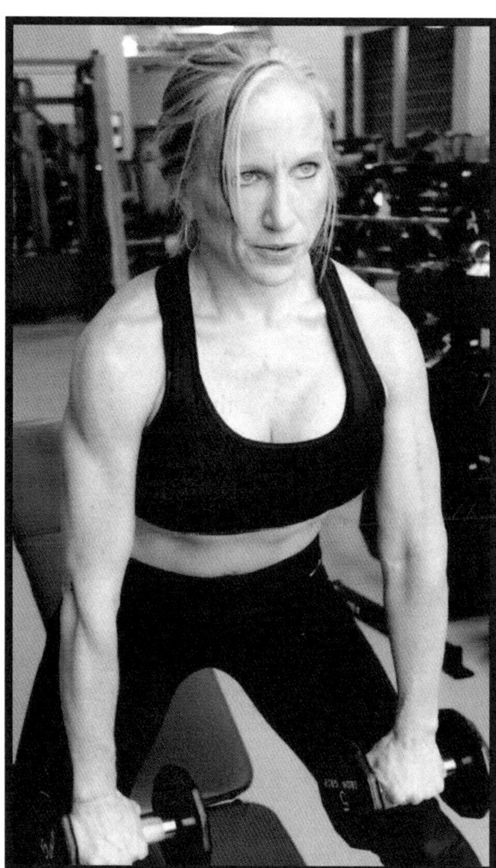

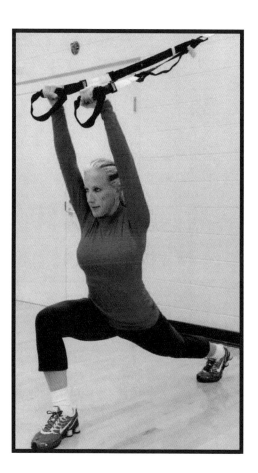

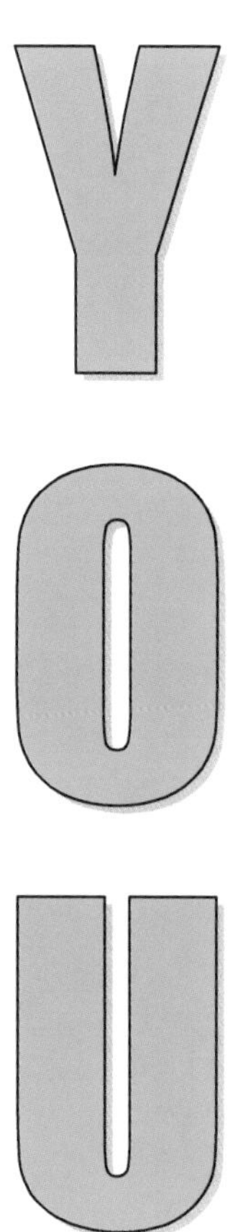

DECIDE

Time for an inspirational sticky note quote, guys. Actually, I have two:

"IT IS NEVER TOO LATE TO BE WHAT YOU MIGHT HAVE BEEN."
—GEORGE ELIOT

"START BY DOING WHAT'S NECESSARY; THEN DO WHAT'S POSSIBLE; AND SUDDENLY YOU ARE DOING THE IMPOSSIBLE."
—ST. FRANCIS OF ASSISI

(Um...WOW. That's it in a brilliant nutshell).

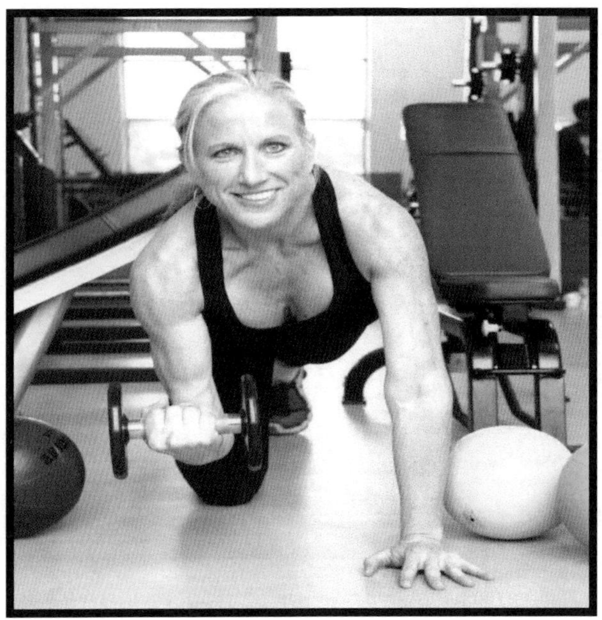

The craziest part about the whole exercise thing is that I almost missed the boat entirely. I know I've already said this, but it bears repeating several (hundred) times. You see…after bariatric surgery, you only have a small window of opportunity to get your you-know-what together. It feels misleading because, like I said you are dropping weight like never before in your life. The danger zone here is that if you do what I almost did, and say SCREW the exercise, you are setting yourself up for failure. I'm telling you (again)…DON'T DO THAT! Exercise is like oxygen...YOU NEED IT! Looking back, it is completely clear (as in crystal) that my window of opportunity to be successful with this surgery was relatively small. You can make or break yourself in the first six to nine months, (at least if you are me). I can't speak for you, because I don't know you. But seriously, I did not go through this surgery and all that has gone before it and along with it only to return to my former state of misery. If I hadn't started exercising, I would have only been marking time.

Physically, a lot has changed since having bariatric surgery. YAY! I lost a whole person! But, CRAP! I had some skin flapping in the wind. My boobs were the worst. Returning them to the northern hemisphere someday was at the top of my "to do" list. Thank God for good sports bras, or I might have knocked myself out during my run. Like I mentioned, my arms and shoulders have been an unexpected, smexy, kruh-mazing, terrifical, magnifitastic transformation. Talk about the HSF! After melting the outer layer of fat away, lookie what was underneath all of that! People are like no freaking way your arms are so ripped. I'm like…WAY. Technically, it's like WHEY, as in protein powder. True, I bust my booty at the gym, but they say abs, arms, etc. are made in the kitchen not in the gym. In my case, I'm a witness to that theory in terms of the muscle definition I've got going on (especially in my upper body). I honestly don't "lift" free weights often. It has everything to do with what I am putting in my body, and for me friends that means P-R-O-T-E-I-N. Good stuff the protein powder is (there's my boy Yoda again). If whey is not for you, there are a bazillion different kinds of protein powders out there. BTW, protein is the building block of muscle...so duh...unless you are allergic or something, drink some! You don't have to spend crazy amounts of casheesh to get it either. At first I thought I had to buy the "bariatric" protein powder. Not true. Those powders are totally fine, but pricey. If you can't afford them (like I couldn't), you have other options. Don't get sucked into the expendiculousness of the protein powder underworld. Last I checked, protein powder needs to have PROTEIN in it. You mix it with water, milk, juice (whatevs), and you drink it. There are different types of protein, and some may have a little extra this or that, but it should be pretty straight forward. Shop it sisters. I get mine in 5-pound containers on Amazon for $50-ish smackeroos (usually with free shipping). Not too shabby, and it lasts me months.

So, what's the deal with all the hanging skin...how much will there be? What can be done about it? Here's my answer. It depends. You'll have to wait and see. Age, gravity, smoking history, and the total amount of weight lost will all determine how much excess skin you are left with. BTW, don't waste your dinero on expensive creams to fix this one. Ain't gonna happen honey. I don't know what your result will be. I know what mine was, and I'll tell you what I did about it.

When you think of the major organs of the human body, the first ones that come to mind are probably the heart, kidneys, and liver. Did you know that skin is the largest organ of the body, making up about 15% of your body's weight? Okay, the human body lesson is over. The point is, we are covered in skin (which is fine) but when the skin is hanging in the wind, well...quite frankly... it's gross (especially when it's hanging on me). One of the bariatric support group meetings I had attended talked about this issue. While it's a quality problem to be at the point where you've lost so much freaking weight that now you have the aesthetics to deal with, it's still a problem. A big old flappy one. Seriously, it can plunge anyone who has experienced massive weight loss into a depression. With the exception of my guns—I mean arms—It made me feel like a skin freak show.

My arms totally throw people for a loop. It's like no one believes that I used to be 300 pounds because I don't have the extra arm skin. Did I get lucky? Not sure, but probably. Okay, I downplay this. Yeah, there's a little luck going on there. I have heard it called "the bat wing," "bingo flappers," or "cafeteria lady arms." Whatever the popular derogatory term...I don't have 'em. I do have a scar on my upper left arm from an old compound fracture 20 years ago, but no surgery otherwise. I didn't dodge the excess skin bullet entirely though. I had the old "bat booty wing" or "booty flapper." Seriously. It looked like someone let all of the air out of my B-hind. Luckily it was nothing a good pair of running pants couldn't squeeze back together. A friend at the gym calls it a "run-on butt." Mine literally had like seven butt chins…I'm not joking (okay, maybe just five). OMG—what's a girl to do?

A reputable plastic surgeon told me:

> "The weight loss and overall improvement in health following bariatric surgery is nothing short of remarkable. Unfortunately, there are significant changes in the skin as elasticity is lost and the skin becomes thinner. The resulting excess skin in various parts of the body can be damaging to your self image as it is a reminder of how you used to be. It is important to be very careful in your selection of a plastic surgeon to help correct these changes. Look for an experienced Plastic Surgeon that is board certified by the American Board of Medical Specialties. This is your assurance that your surgeon has completed rigorous training, certification and re-certification. Also confirm your selection by asking your primary care physician, friends or family that have had plastic surgery, or hospital staff that are knowledgeable about the doctor you are considering.
>
> I tell my patients that are considering plastic surgery while they are seeking a weight loss goal, that they should be near their goal prior to proceeding. I also reinforce that diet alone is rarely the solution to weight loss, just as bariatric surgery alone is rarely successful in the long term. Regular exercise is vital for both health maintenance and long term success in weight loss".
>
> --Dr. John Aker

Everything you need is already inside. Just do it.
—Bill Bowerman, Nike

(BTW, Nike…I think I love you, and I don't care who knows it.
Thanks for making a smexy running shoe in a size 11).

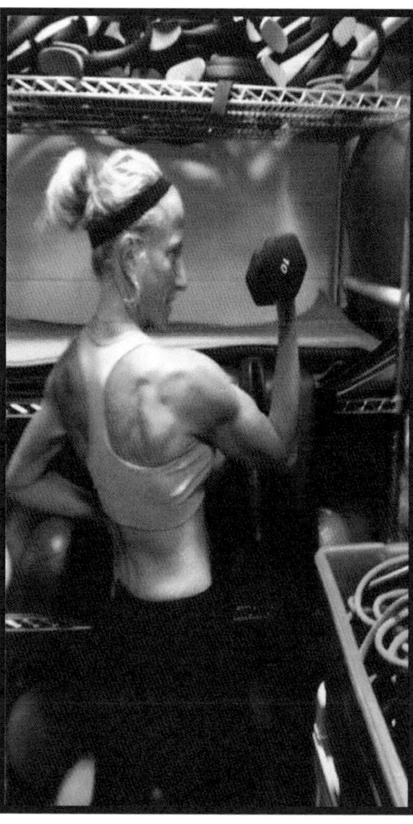

Expurthit's in size 11

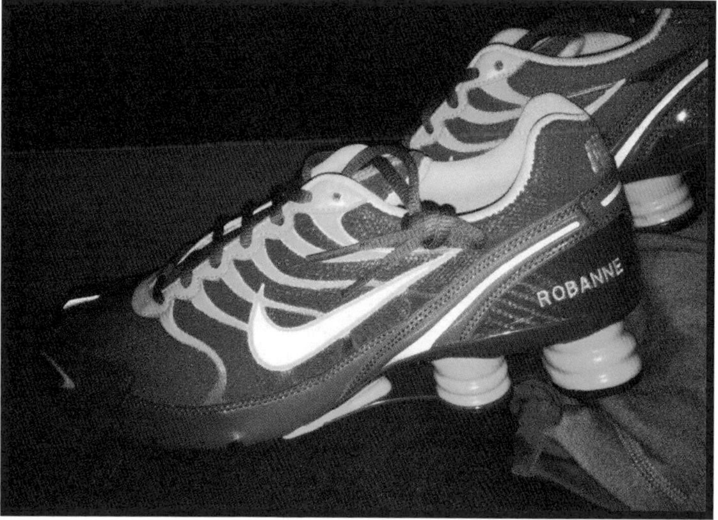

I read somewhere that your ears, nose and feet grow your entire life. YIPPEE! I should be a Pinochio-Dumbo hybrid on skis in a few more years. I'm not worried…as long as there's a swoosh on them, I'll be o.k.

AUGUST 2000

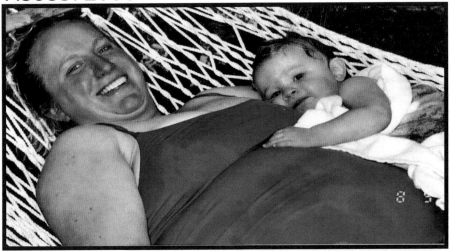

impossible = i'm possible!

OCTOBER 2012

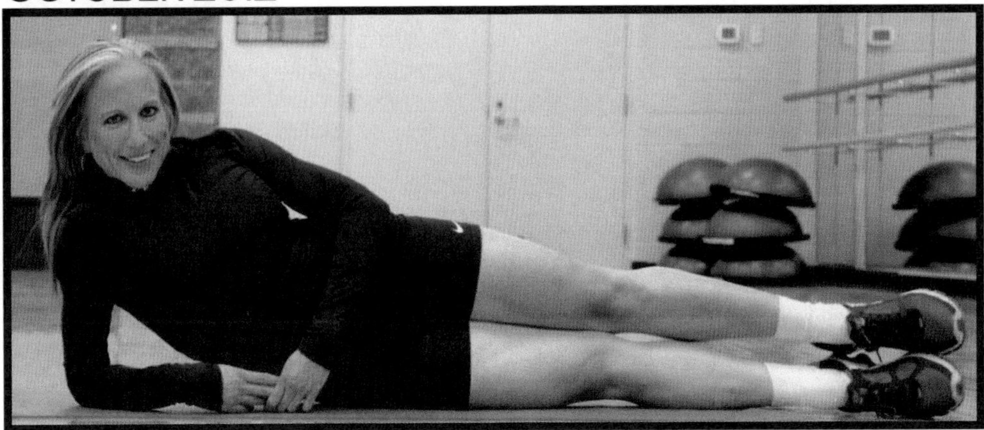

Warning - If you skipped ahead to this chapter because the extra skin mystery is killing you, I can't say that I blame you (cheater). I can also tell you that I don't solve this Scooby-Doo skin mystery either, so don't get your hopes up. For real though, you should go back and read the first 9 chapters.

10

Sporks

Honestly, when it comes to excess skin and SAG, you don't have to have dropped a massive amount of weight to know what I am talking about. I think most, if not all women experience "the sag" as they age, and as gravity opens up a grade-A can of whoop-ass on them. If you've given birth and breast-fed children…then you really know what I am talking about.

Now, I repeat, EVERYONE is different with the skin business. What's sagging and dragging on me when the weight came off may be riding high on you. My life experience is like the excess skin trifecta. It has included having three children and breast feeding, having age and gravity work their magic on me, and experiencing massive weight loss. I was "lucky" enough to have the saggy girls, the old muffin top/wiggle-jiggle tummy, slappy thighs and booty drag. I don't care how you lose your weight, or even how much you lose…you just don't feel like a smexy, attractive woman with wrinkly, shriveled-up boobs and butt to match.

When I looked at my chest, I felt like I was looking at hanging tube socks. Now please don't take what I'm about to say the wrong way. I'm not a basher of anything, and I'm not about to buck that trend and start ripping on tribal females, but it's the most clear-cut visual I can give you, without actually showing you. You could have slapped a nose ring on me and put me on the cover of National Geographic with how low the "girls" were hanging. It was hard for me to look at all that saggy, draping skin. It reminded me of every pound of fat that I couldn't stand. I get why people who lose a ton of weight get very depressed. It's like you resent yourself for doing that to your body in the first place coupled with just being plain old PO'd at gravity. Every stretched out ounce of skin stares back at you and it's ugg-lee. Think about it, once you deflate a 300-pound balloon to half its size, you are left with a lot of "sag". Having been there, it's almost as depressing as weighing 300 pounds.

On a lighter note, Webster's is just cracking me up. Look up "sag." Here, I'll do it for you. It reads: "a part or area that sinks or hangs below the natural or right level." You could say that again sister! I had a few "areas" that fit that description. Thank God for good plastic surgeons and oodles of overtime where I work so I could afford to have it removed. I know you are probably freaking out about paying for something that is at the very least a year away for you. Pump the brakes. You can save up like I did, or there are financing options. Trust that where there is a will (and hopefully some overtime), there is a way. The majority of people I know who have had skin removed have had to plunk down the dinero to do it. But, long shot as it may be, your insurance may help out with it (but don't count on it). Just being honest.

I really thought I would be happy enough just having lost the weight. I would have never told you I would EVER have plastic surgery, until I experienced what it was like to have all of that hanging skin. Here's what I needed to do for me: I had plastic surgery on my tummy, outer thighs and buns to remove excess skin. I also had my tatas done. Ba-bye tube socks. Hello spork boobies. What? Don't worry. I'm about to explain. Let's just say plastic surgery number one was a disaster. I ended up having all of it re-done by another surgeon to fix everything. That was an expendiculously dangerous lesson.

We'll call surgery #1 "the plastic disaster". At my two-week post-op check-up, things were tight and pulled really easy (fairly normal, so far so good). I could barely sit down to pee let alone stand up straight. I had boobs, but they were not right. They were big (which is what I wanted), but they sagged at the bottom (not O.K., definitely NOT O.K.). I was told they would "drop into the pocket." Whatever the heck that meant? Basically, that's code for: your surgeon should have done a mastopexy to remove all of the excess skin.

Mastopexy MASS-toh-pex-ee:
cosmetic surgery intended to lift the breast and nipple/areola to a higher, more youthful position.
English translation: putting the "girls" back in the Northern Hemisphere where they belong.

I had implants put in, but no mastopexy the first time around. BIG MISTAKE. I was misguided by a plastic surgeon whose name doesn't bare repeating (not to mention, I'll get sued). Now instead of the previously saggy, limited edition National Geographic boobies, I had what I called "spork boobs". Not sure why I called them that other than they were freak-show-alienesque, like I was a regular at that cantina all the creatures in Stars Wars go to. Just when I didn't think my boobs could look any freakier, I had basically exchanged tube socks for sporks. Not exactly the upgrade I was going for. The sporks were more of an expendonculous lateral move. Now, I don't really want to show you my gross spork boobies so I won't. But suffice to say they were creepy-gross. Good news is plastic surgery #2 went very well (we'll call that one "the plastic fantastic"). Since having them re-done, they went from freak-show to fabulous...and sorry Charlie, you can't see them either. Although I contemplated adding them in so you can get that tube sock-spork boob visual out of your head. (Sorry, hope I didn't scar you). But if you're not afraid and want to see the whole sha-bang including scars, sporks and all (and you know you do), there is a full monty supplement to this book appropriately entitled "Sag" you can check out. We'll talk later. Time for a quick public service announcement—if you are considering having "the girls" done, get a mammogram before you go messing around with things. If the plastic surgeon you are considering doesn't require one (RED FLAG), then go to one that does.

Anyway, after all that plastic surgery, from a fitness standpoint, my 7 and a ½ minute, uphill mile regressed to a 30 minute walking mile. I was getting passed right and left by crawling babies and silver sneakers. Patience was my biggest challenge. I would have never imagined ever complaining that I couldn't exercise. HOLY CRAPPITS life has changed! Seriously, these days I would need therapy if I couldn't exercise! (I might still need it anyway, but especially if I couldn't exercise). I had to listen to my doctor, my trainer, and my body and do what was right. That included backing off on the hip hop classes for a few months (GASP). Anyhoo, over the next several months I was able to slowly work my way back up to my usual workout groove. Post snip, nip and tuck I've made some changes to adapt to the new landscape. Guess what…if something feels funny, or pulls too much…I stop (what a concept).

Now what about sex? Well now...this has been interesting. Prior to my surgery my husband and I went through very long periods without sex—six to nine months sometimes. I mean like nada enchilada, as in zero, zilch, absolute bupkis. Food was my boyfriend. It's all I wanted, and it didn't care how I looked. I would pass out every night in a self-induced food coma. I had to satisfy my cravings for pasta, or chocolate cake, or whatever. So safe to say, there wasn't a lot of nookie. Not to mention...have you tried sex at 300 pounds? Not so easy, and you feel embarrassed doing it. Even if you can find the energy, you're out of breath before you get started, and mortified the entire time watching all of your fat folds slosh around. It's kind of hard to get into it when you feel that much shame and disgust for yourself. On top of that, you know that your partner has to be thinking something along those lines. So on the (very) few occasions we dared attempt "relations," lights were out and lots of clothes were left on so I wouldn't have to see so much of what I was…so much of me that I couldn't get rid of...so much of me that I was stuck in. I was trapped in this body that I didn't want anymore, and hadn't wanted for years, but I couldn't find my way out. How do you live not wanting to be fat, but not being able to stop the insanity that has deteriorated to indifference? I was in that spot and it sucked. I mean S-U-C-K sucked. If you are in that spot, I hope it sucks for you too. I know that sounds very insensitive and quite possibly just flat-out mean. But let's be honest. You're not going to change unless you are in that spot, right? And if you're like me, you'll also need two fun-filled trips to the ER before you take action.

Since the weight loss, my marriage has had its issues. I feel like I have made huge changes, and gotten kruh-mazing results. There are times when my husband, who can admittedly be Mr. Fatty McButterpants, isn't taking care of himself. I found that I was encouraging him to exercise and eat right. Frustrating. It reminds me of the position I put him in for a decade. Having to watch his spouse eat herself into oblivion, and for the most part live as platonic roommates, because we just didn't have sex. Having lost the weight and having the skin removed I feel really good about my body. Now the clothes can come off and the lights can stay on (sorry TMI). We aren't swinging from the chandelier or anything, but today, we motivate each other and love and life are back in business (but just for the record, I'm in better shape).

As for clothes and shopping, oh…don't get me started! Do you have any idea how freaking AWESOME it is to go shopping now?! I still get giddy just thinking about it. I wear a 6 or an 8…my former size used to have a "2" in front of that number (26 or 28), and there was always a letter after the size like "W" or "X." I have worn a 3X-4X before and a 26W-28W. Even elastic waistbands were tight at times…not to mention the granny panties. Try getting those bad boys out of a bunch! It's so exciting to go shopping for sassy bathing suits. For over a decade I have dreaded the thought of wearing a bathing suit. I have gone from the moo-moo mom-kini to a bikini! STFD, girlfriend! WTH!!! I remember several summers ago, I must have lost another bet or something because I went to the pool in a bathing suit. Anyhoo, there were like five moms in the same plus-size Target bathing suit/cover-up/hybrid-contraption—I was one of them. Let's just say, I came in a distant 5th in the "looking good, rocking it out" department. I just wanted to go drown myself (O.K., perhaps a bit dramatic). I just wanted to go under the water up to my neck. Back then I wanted to be invisible which meant my kids missed out on me participating in physical activities. Now it's totally different! I won't be hitting a nude beach anytime soon (or probably ever), but I enjoy going to the pool now and swimming with the kids. I still have parts of my bod that are a little jiggly, but I'll take it. Interestingly enough, for months after hitting my goal weight I would still go on auto-pilot when I went shopping and naturally gravitate to the "Woman's World" section. It was like a pre-programmed cruise control setting I couldn't clear. Even having lost all that weight, it took an entire year to get used to the idea I could shop in a section that didn't have the word "plus" or "world" in it.

2008

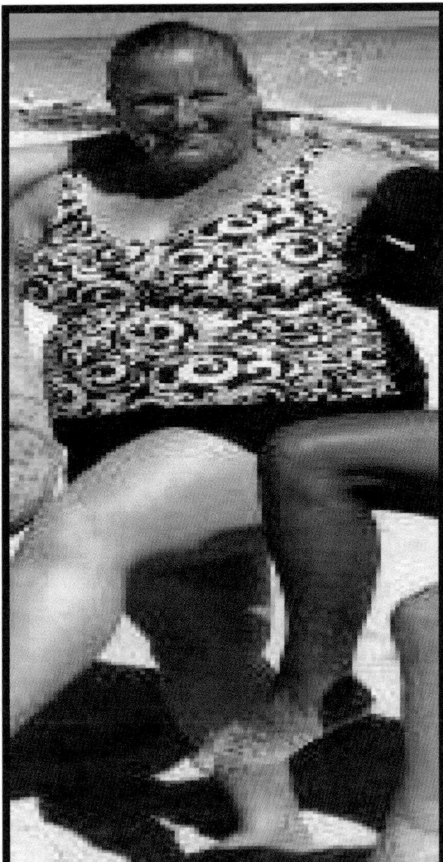

This would be the award winning plus-size moo-moo, mom-kini, hybrid contraption I speak of.

2012

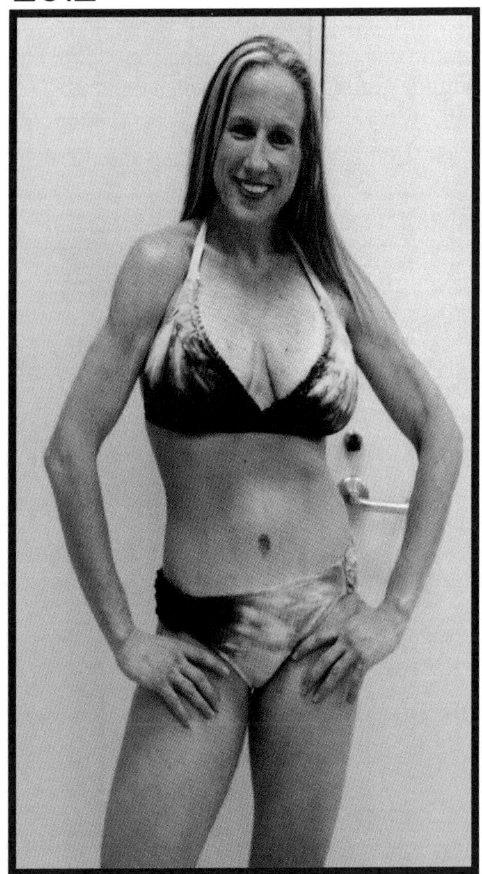

Holy crappits—I'm in a bikini (and not because I lost a bet).

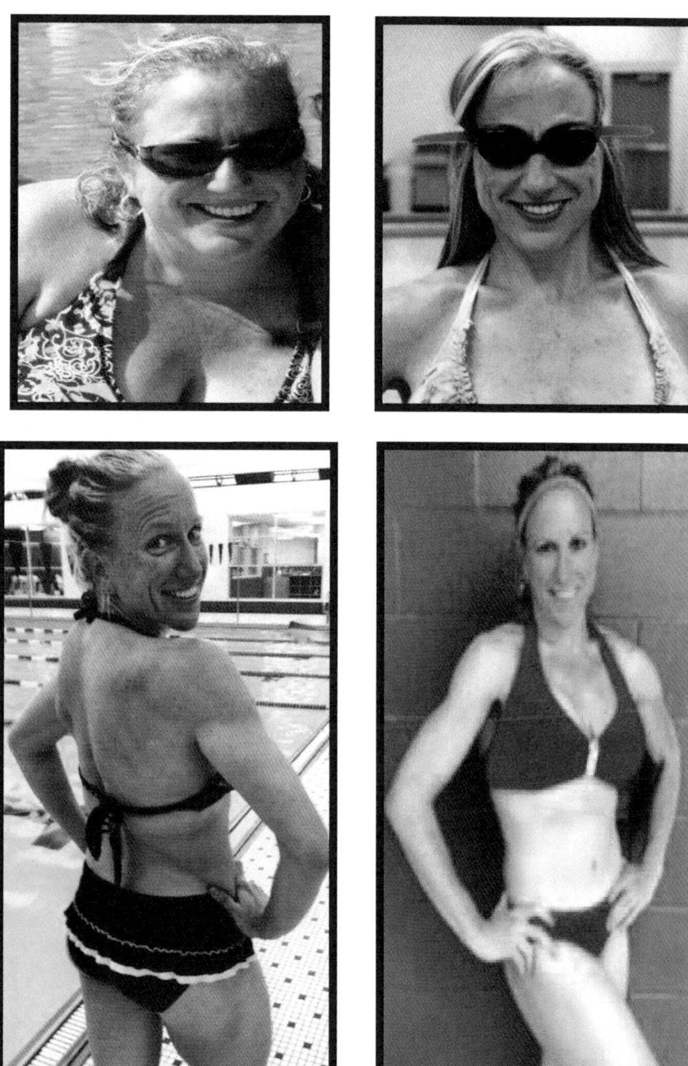

I'm not all that and a bag of baked chips or anything, but this whole bikini situation is nothing short of winning the weight loss lottery…twice. Not sure I'll ever *not* be amazed. BTW, my stomach hasn't seen the sun in a decade, hence I am as white as Wonder bread. I'm also Lithuanian. My people don't tan and we have giant pores. AWESOME. Look out! Here comes another PSA…like a cigarette is to the lung, tanning beds are to the skin—CANCER CAUSING. I don't care if you glow in the dark—stay the heck away from them! And for the love of God, put some sunscreen on. Sheesh…don't know where all that came from, but apparently the nurse in me needed to say it. And, you're still getting the mammogram we talked about earlier.

It's really kruh-mazing to be able to go into a store, shop off of the regular size racks, and have stuff fit. I can still remember grabbing a size 6 or 8 and bringing it into the fitting room in fear of trying it on. I just couldn't believe that size was going to fit me! It did, and now I know that it will. Maybe that fear comes from all of the times I tried on clothes in the biggest size they had with no luck Chuck? I remember toward the end of my obese road, I only bought my elastic-waisted, plus-size mom jeans at Wal-Mart or Target off the full-figured clearance racks. D-to-the-pressing! Although, migrating from the superstore clearance racks to the fun stuff is how I came up with the words expendiculous, expurthit, and expendeccessary. (Maybe I'll hit expendonculous if this book sells). Okay, I said I wouldn't help you, but that's four made-up words in a row. Please turn to the glossary at the front of the book for translation.

Some kruh-mazing comments people have made to me: Last summer when I was getting off the plane in Orange County, CA (hottie central, USA) the flight attendant customarily saying "ba-bye" to everyone as they deplane, says to me, "Oh, you must be here for the fitness convention." I looked over my shoulder, (and it became apparent she was talking to me). STFD and the back door too! I don't think I stopped smiling for the rest of the day. Another time, someone asked me if I was a fitness guru, and another time someone said..."Are you here for the race?" Does it get any better than that? Well, actually it does. I was at a Hip Hop Hustle certification recently and a lady asked me if I was the director of the event...the freaking director!!! It was like I died and went to hip hop heaven.

To the contrary, I have had many people who knew 300-pound me take it upon themselves to look after me. They let me know that I am "wasting away," and that I should not lose another ounce. I remind myself of the facts Jack…I weigh 150 pounds, I am 5'7 ('ish). I am fine, certainly nowhere near too thin, and I've maintained this weight in a healthy manner for over a year and a half. I've shown you what the Skeletor Robanne and 300-pound Robanne looked like. Yeah, not there anymore.

Then there are those that say, "You didn't need to have bariatric surgery." I have been told that I could have lost the weight on my own. Okay...really? (That's good to know—why didn't I think of that one?) If I could have, I would have! Bariatric surgery was an absolute last resort. It was the tool I needed to turn things 180 ° from hot mess to healthy. Oh, and this one's my fave: "Why couldn't you have just followed the bariatric diet plan without having the surgery?" For real, people! AYFKM? I take a deep breath, and say, "Well, it's a little something called HUNGER!" When your stomach is bariatric size (2-5'ish ounces), it's possible to follow the bariatric food plan. Without having the surgery, it would be like me asking you to drink a little chicken broth, and a sip of juice and call that your meal. Not possible. You'd be gnawing your arm off by lunch time. It is a quality problem to even be fielding these comments (seriously). But, offering unsolicited advice on someone's life-or-death issues is a ballsy move, not to mention potentially hazardous. They have no idea they could be saying something detrimental as all get out. So I consider the source. If "they" lack clinical background or personal experience to back up their expert commentary, I dismiss it. I hope I am not sounding like that guy. I'll be the first to say, I don't know what's best for you, but I do have my own experience to share. Take what you can use, ask professionals lots of questions, and leave the rest behind.

So how does this story end? It doesn't really. I don't beat myself up over it, but I am acutely aware that I will always referee food and my 300-pound brain. On a daily basis, I remind myself what I am capable of...and it's 300 pounds of scary. Actually, it would probably be worse. If I return to my old behaviors, I would very likely pick up where I left off, and go downhill from there. I have seen many a bariatric patient lose a ton of weight...and then slap it all right back on. One last time for the road...just like any type of weight loss, bariatric surgery is a tool to aid in weight loss. It enabled me to get my mojo moving in the right direction for the first time in years, but it is by no means a permanent fix. In order to cross over into the land of long-term results, lifestyle change must occur.

-Change occurs when Inspiration and Motivation meet Perspiration-

I blurted that out one day and I totally believe it. I live it. Here we go with Dr. Phil again...I'm paraphrasing, but I'm pretty sure he would say..."God will move mountains, but you better show up with a wheelbarrow." I bring my wheelbarrow every damn day and do my part of the deal, plain and simple.

Here's my dealio. I work out five days a week and eat small meals throughout the day. I choose protein over carbs, although I don't agree with giving up carbs. My body needs them; it just doesn't need the two plates of pasta or white rice kind of carbs that I used to glom on all the time. Now, I go for whole grain carbs, and I start every day with oatmeal (no sugar added). Exercise has saved me. It's my secret weapon, and it not only helped get me in shape, <u>it keeps me here</u> (now there's a neat trick). It has given me the strength and endurance I thought I would never have. Amazing to be fit it is (thanks Yoda). I am not sure what to say to those of you who cannot exercise either by choice, or by circumstance, other than to say that I am concerned for your long-term success if you don't adopt a healthy physical exercise program. Seriously, it's about changing EVERYTHING. I used to never exercise, short of having to run for my life...in which case, I would be dead by now.

DON'T LET WHAT YOU CANNOT DO INTERFERE WITH WHAT YOU CAN DO
—JOHN WOODEN

Here it is again...

Clean version:

-ASK YOUR DOCTOR IF GETTING OFF YOUR BUTT IS RIGHT FOR YOU-

Explicit version:

-ASK YOUR DOCTOR IF GETTING OFF YOUR A$$ IS RIGHT FOR YOU-

Today, I am no longer a bystander in my own life. Not only can I fully participate in the lives of my children, I can catch them if they try and make a break for it. We run, we play, we ride bikes, and guess what...we go to the pool, and I rock a bikini these days. By "rock" I mean I am 40 ('ish) and have lost half my body weight, and was fortunate enough to find a talented plastic surgeon the second time. I am an example of healthy living today. For that, I am truly grateful. You couldn't have told me three years after having bariatric surgery I would write this book and share my story to inspire and motivate others. After eating myself to death for a decade, and starving myself and puking my guts out for years before that, I had all but given up on ever finding some sense of normalcy in the food/weight/healthy lifestyle department. I had certainly given up on ever getting out of that body I was trapped in. I was convinced I was going to be 300-pound me forever. When I began this process, getting fit and strong weren't on my to-do list, either. I was just focused on losing the weight, and watching the numbers on the scale go down. Then things changed.

As the fat began to melt away, and the muscles came out to play—my focus shifted to being STRONG and FIT! I finally got it. It's not just about losing weight. It's so much more than that. My purpose today is sharing my story and inspiring others to reach for their STRONG. Everyone's got a challenge (or two) to overcome. As I have dished up, mine included eating disorders and gastric bypass surgery—starting with childhood obesity, followed by anorexia and bulimia, then morbid obesity, and bariatric surgery. It's no surprise that having a healthy body image has been a major hurdle for me. Being skinny is great if it's not "fake skinny." My quest for skinny got me way off track long ago. If there is anything I want to let young ladies out there know (and young men too, but ESPECIALLY the young ladies), it is that...

SKINNY IS OVERRATED! SO GET YOUR STRONG ON!

strong

healthy, having powerful action or effect

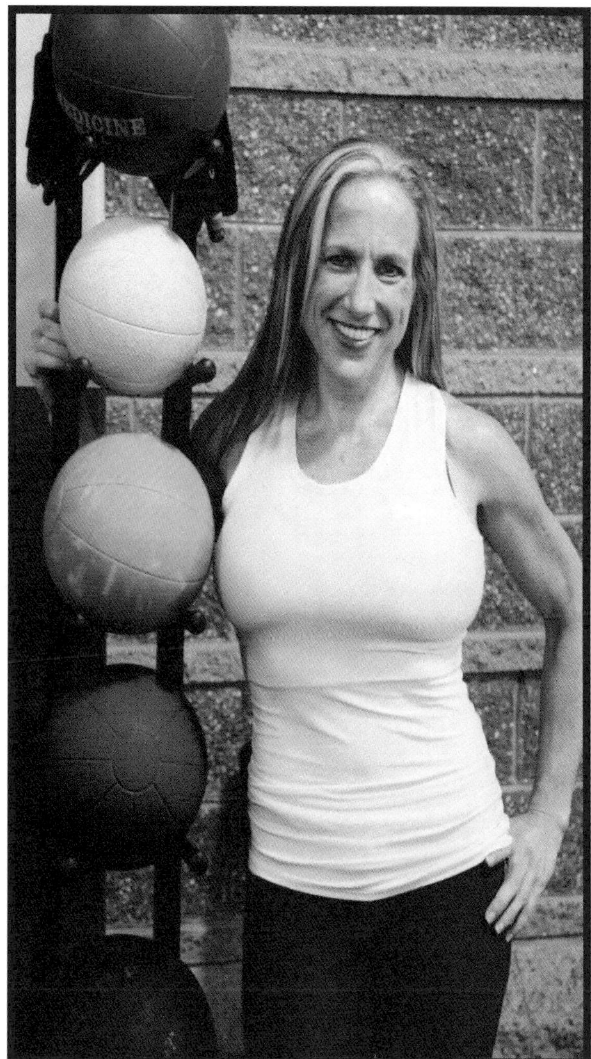

October 2012

BE STRONG

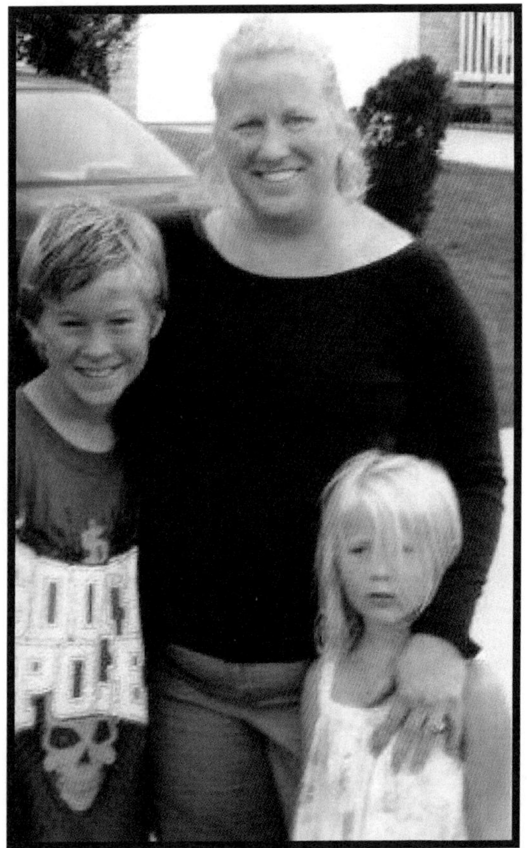

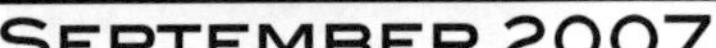

SEPTEMBER 2007

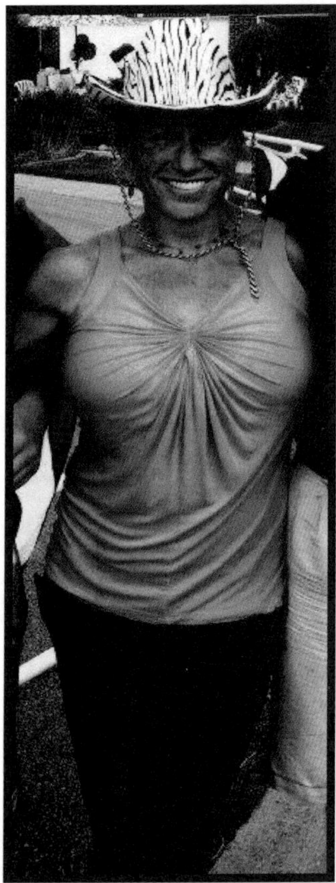

AUGUST 2012

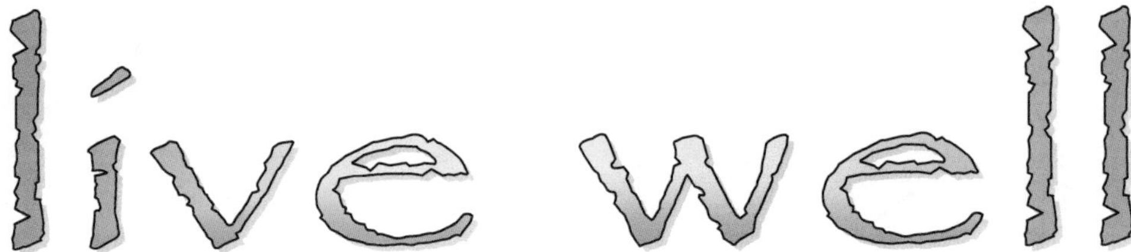

11

Get Your STRONG On!

It's not about being thin...it's just not! Today, my passion is to promote the message to our young people the value of being STRONG. We've gone from the "clean your plate" generation to the "size double-zero skinny jeans" generation. I don't know which I despise more.

It's not the size of your jeans; it's not the number on the scale. Health and fitness has no exact, pre-determined size, no exact weight. It shows itself in many ways, and what's right for me may be way off for you. I find it concerning that even revealing my weight of 150 pounds takes people aback. We are so pre-programmed to weigh less, the smaller the number the better, right? NOT! Why is 150 pounds too much for some people to hear? I know I am healthy at that weight which is really all that matters. Having been anorexic and bulimic, it fires me up when I get feedback like..."there's no way you can weigh 150...you look more like 125." Or, there's the..."well, muscle weighs more than fat" as if to justify and excuse my weight. That can really mess with a food addict's head. These statements are contradictory, considering a few pages back "they" were ready to force feed me a cheeseburger. Rather than let "them" make up their minds, I made up mine. My doctors would agree, I'm the healthiest Robanne I have ever been. And so it is.

-STRONG IS THE NEW SKINNY-

Girls and boys (especially our adolescent and tweenie/teenies)...I'm talking to you, so listen up! You are perfectly fine NOT weighing 100 pounds soaking wet out of the shower. Forbid yourself from comparing yourself to others. I always tried to justify weighing 115 pounds at 5'7 ('ish) because I knew the 5-foot girls weighed about a buck o' five. That's just messed up thinking. A healthy body has different weights based on height and muscle mass, plain and simple. Stop comparing how inadequate you may feel on the inside to how good someone looks on the outside. Trust me sisters, it's not a fair fight. I got handed a royal butt whooping every time.

Today I strive for balance. Not sure I'll ever get there, but it's fun trying. I'm pretty sure I'll always do too much of something, I just try to make it a "good" something. Exercise and nourishment are top priorities. I moved myself from the bottom of the list to the tippity-top. As hard as it can be at times, I consciously take the actions to fit myself into my own damn life. Why is that so hard? But it is! It sounds silly to even say it, but how many of us are too busy to make time for ourselves, too busy to workout, or pack a healthy lunch? Well, I call bull honkey on that, sisters. If I can do it, so can you. After all, you can't take care of others if you don't take care of yourself. Can I get another Amen?

I'm no David Letterman, but I do have a top 10 list.
The top 10 things I do to stay on track are: (drum roll please)

1. I AM HONEST WITH MYSELF. No more B.S., no more excuses, no more Splenda-coated rationalizations. That ship has sailed. It's time for the straight-up truth so I don't return to 300-pound me. I am honest at every meal, and I stay far, far away from all-you-can-eat buffets, drive-thrus and French fries. On a daily basis, I acknowledge that I am a bariatric patient, and therefore need to behave like one.

2. I DON'T PROCRASTINATE. I do what I say I'm going to do, when I say I'm going to do it (unless of course, I'm injured, sick, or dead. In which case, I can't do it).

3. I HAVE HIGH HOPES AND, (with the help of others), REASONABLE EXPECTATIONS. I am an optimist (with an occasional flair for the depressive side). So having said that, it is ultra important not to set myself up for failure by setting unattainable goals. Often times, I am not the best one to figure out what is "reasonable." In fact, I'm pretty sure I suck at that when it comes to me, but, the good news is I know people who are tremendous at it (doctors, hip hop gurus, and one heck of an amazing PT). I call them my "A-team". Get one. BTW, when it comes to figuring out what's reasonable for my husband—I'm awesome at it.

4. I HAVE A HEALTHY PERSPECTIVE (more often than not these days). Let's see what Webster's has to say about perspective. Ahh...definition #3… "the ability to understand what is important and what isn't". The majority of my life I was pretty lost with a few things. Today I am clear on what matters, but I have found from time to (depressive) time that I need to speak with a shrink (to do something other than obtain a signature). Asking for help has never been my forte, but neither has having a healthy perspective.

5. I PREPARE FOR SUCCESS. I set myself up for success rather than failure by taking the time for me to prepare things ahead of time. I make sure to surround myself with healthy choices. If you do that, I have found chances are you will actually make them. Dare to prepare (and that may mean toting around a cooler). And while you're at it—pack your gym clothes the night before and have them ready to go! Thanks to directions from my PT, I keep an extra set of gym clothes in the trunk of my car. That way I can never conger up the excuse that I don't have what I need to go exercise. Evil genius.

6. I KEEP AT IT. There is no try, only do (what's up Yoda). I set meals and my workouts up (in advance). I know what food is in my fridge and when I'm working out (what days, times, classes, PT sessions, etc.). I write them on my calendar and actually show up to them. I call dibs on some "me time" and it doesn't get bumped for anything (unless their last name is Robin and they are bleeding or on fire or something).

7. I AM DETERMINED YET FLEXIBLE. I know what I want. But like the Rolling Stones have sung, "You can't always get what you want...but if you try sometimes...you just might get what you need." I trust in the process. I worry less and chill more, and it usually works out just fine and dandy.

8. I LEARN FROM MY PAST. There is huge value in failure. My lifetime of eating disorders is quite frankly one of my best assets. It is a great motivator to stay exactly the heck where I am. Just in case I wake up stupid, I use my sticky note quotes (figuratively), and it never hurts to stick a picture of 300-pound me smack dab next to 150-pound me. That's a no-brainer, friends.

9. I MAKE TIME FOR ME. (again) This is kind of like #6, but I put it in again with a pampering twist this time. If you are like I was, you suck at making time for yourself. (So "you time" needs to be highlighted). MVM'S across the land... put the kiddos somewhere safe and give yourself the gift of taking care of yourself so you in turn can take (better) care of them. They would want you to do that (unless of course they are toddlers, in which case they would rather have you chase them around all day, helping them to avoid certain dangers that they have an uncanny knack for finding).

10. I HAVE A BLAST. I have decided I am going to be with myself all day anyway, so I might as well make it enjoyable (those around me like this idea too). I take chances and step out of my comfy zone on a regular basis, and that has proven to be quite the adventure for this serial creature of habit. I also occasionally wear a super hero costume to the wellness center (no lie).

make today ridiculously amazing

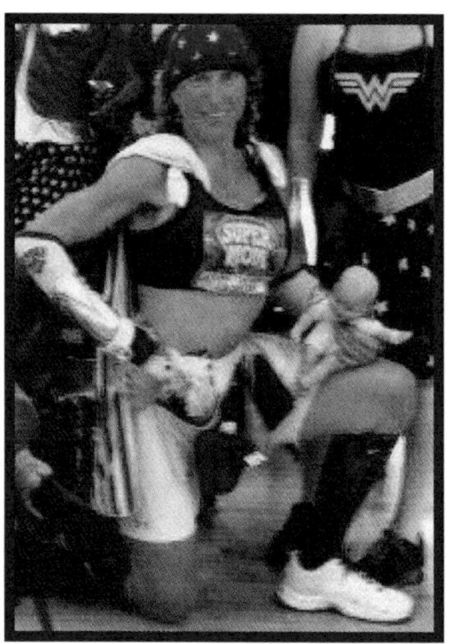

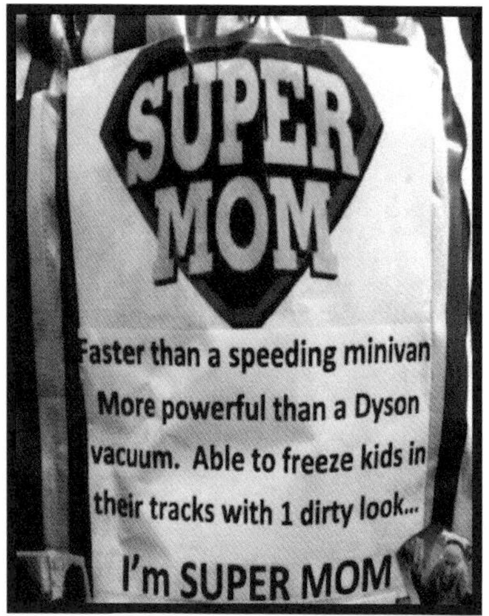
SUPER
MOM
Faster than a speeding minivan
More powerful than a Dyson
vacuum. Able to freeze kids in
their tracks with 1 dirty look...
I'm SUPER MOM

LIVING THE MINIVAN DREAM

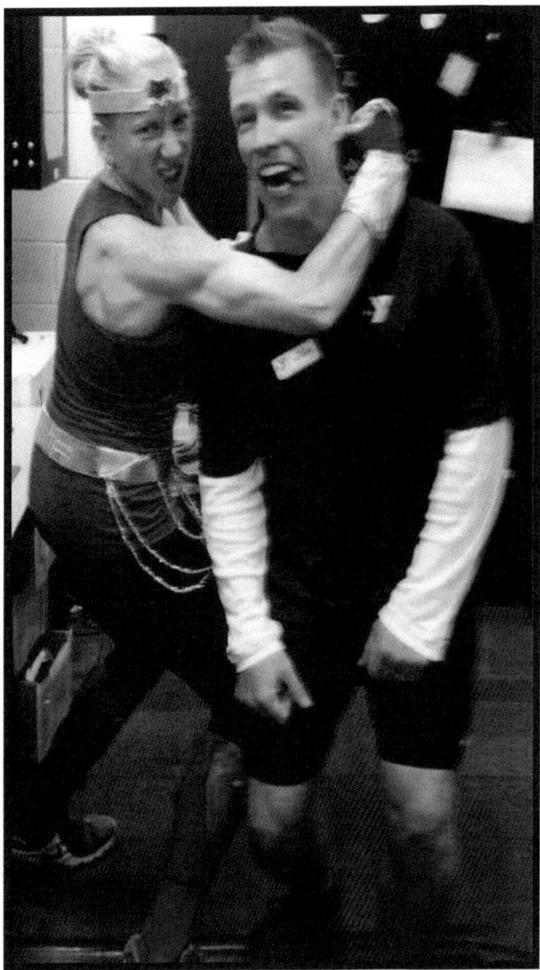

With Matt Newmann, A.C.S.M., C.P.T.

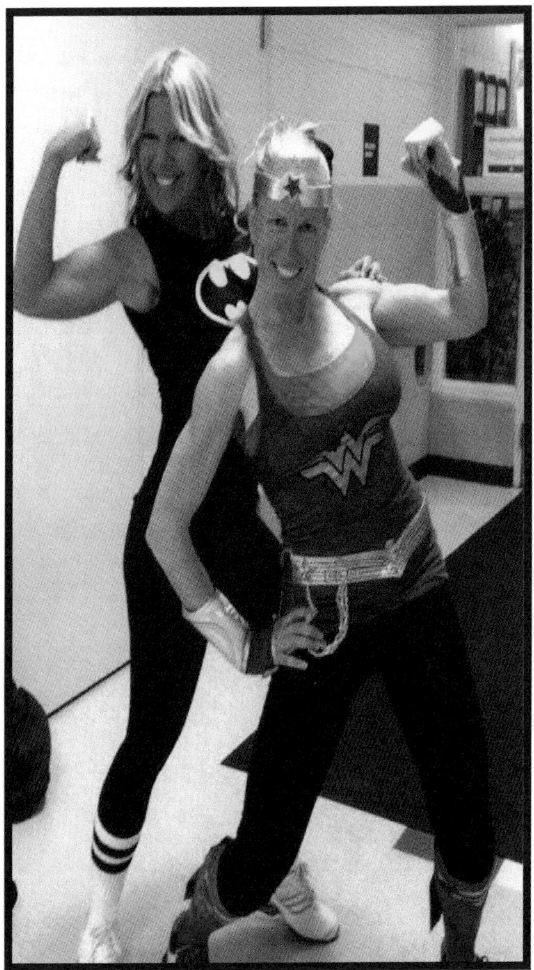

With Hip Hop Hustle Instructor, Denise Mirro

I DON'T TRUST ANYONE WHO DOESN'T LAUGH
—MAYA ANGELOU

Luck is the byproduct of preparation. So, I wish you "luck" on your situation, whatever it is. If you share my struggle with weight, eating disorders, and body image I want to spread the message I heard loud and clear on the radio that nippy November day. No matter how you achieve your weight loss, you will not be able to maintain it unless you change your lifestyle. What started out as a journey to lose weight and make it off the couch has become an odyssey that has launched me into STRONG. Because, although this has been one heck of a ride, it's not truly a journey. A journey implies an end – the act of traveling from one place to another. An odyssey, on the other hand, is an extended adventurous trip or voyage. I'll take door #2, thank you. Who knows where I will go from here and where Getting My STRONG On will take me and hopefully others?

NEVER give up on you. NEVER.
I almost did, and look what's happening to me!

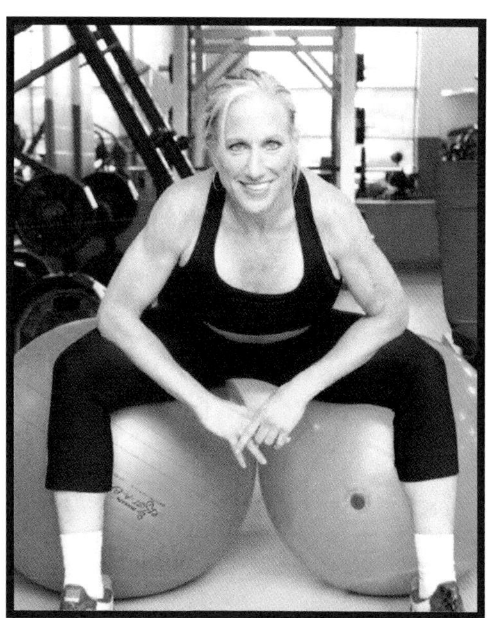

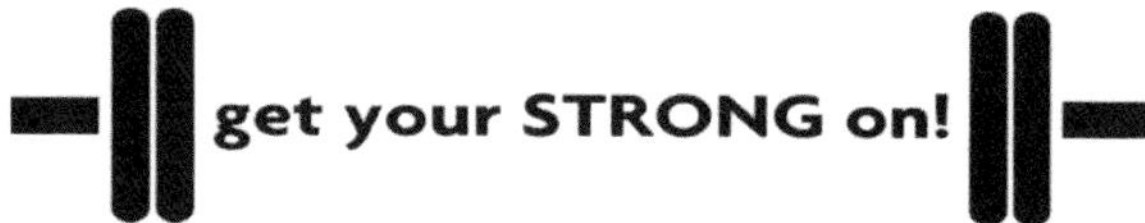

Hope

is like peace.
It is not a gift from God.
It is a gift only we can
give one another.

-Elie Wiesel

12
The "Other Stuff"

Anyone who doesn't have "other stuff" to sort out in this life is either on some really good medication, or lying. At certain points in my life, I've been both medicated or lying. On a really rough day, I've been a medicated liar. There are two things I am certain of— first, that I'll always be sorting out some kind of "stuff", and second, just when I think the previously sorted out stuff is handled…POOF…it tries to sneak its way back in, or even sneakier, it reappears in some other fashion.

For anyone reading this that struggles with depression (like girlfriend over here), do yourself a HUGE solid and go talk to someone. Get some help. SERIOUSLY. My eating disorders and depression were completely intertwined. On more than one occasion, I have found it necessary to see a counselor, therapist, psychologist, or psychiatrist. I can easily get off track if I become my own air traffic controller. Even after the weight loss, I still have the same (often chemically imbalanced) brain that I had before. (Although now, I pretty much think life rocks). However, my expectations of myself are often too high and I can easily set myself up for disappointment and shift depression into overdrive. I have found it invaluable to run my thinking by someone else more qualified than me to sort it out. Professionals are amazing at this since they are (unlike my husband or girlfriends) fairly objective. For me, treating my "other stuff" has meant taking medication (GASP). In the past, I got really hung up on this. It's harder than heck for me to admit I need more help than I've already got going. But, I've gotten over myself (thank God). I mean, if I were diabetic, I would be o.k. taking insulin, so why is treating my brain any different? I share this with you not because I want to steer you toward medication. That's not my call. What I want to stress is that it's O.K. to need help. You don't want to be so self-sufficient that you get to where I was—literally trying to punch my own ticket with food everyday and in between bites day dreaming about how easy it would be to drive my car off a cliff or something. In this voyage of mine, I have had to not only address diet and exercise, but to face emotional and psychological issues. In the words of someone much more qualified than me to handle "my stuff", here goes:

"Life happens around us and the best way to have a good one is finding the balance in your life. The brain is an organ that we have been ignoring for far too long. It's time to let go of the stigma and take care of ourselves and our children so the emotional struggle does not become a limiting factor in our lives".

—Muhammad T. Munir, M.D.

Dr. Munir completed his residency in adult psychiatry at Wayne State School of Medicine in Michigan, followed by a fellowship in child and family psychiatry at Brown University in Rhode Island.

HOLY *MOLY PHOTO GALLERY

Here are more before and after photos that I never dreamed possible. When I began this transformation, I had no clue I was headed for STRONG. I was just hoping to lose enough weight to make it up the stairs without becoming short of breath. I got a heck of a lot more out of the deal.

*BTW, according to Wikipedia, "moly" may refer to a magic herb in Greek mythology, or a type of flowering plant. Phew! It's a good thing we don't have to say "holy mythical magic Greek herb" every time we have a "holy moly" situation. That would be a mouthful. "Moly" will work just fine.

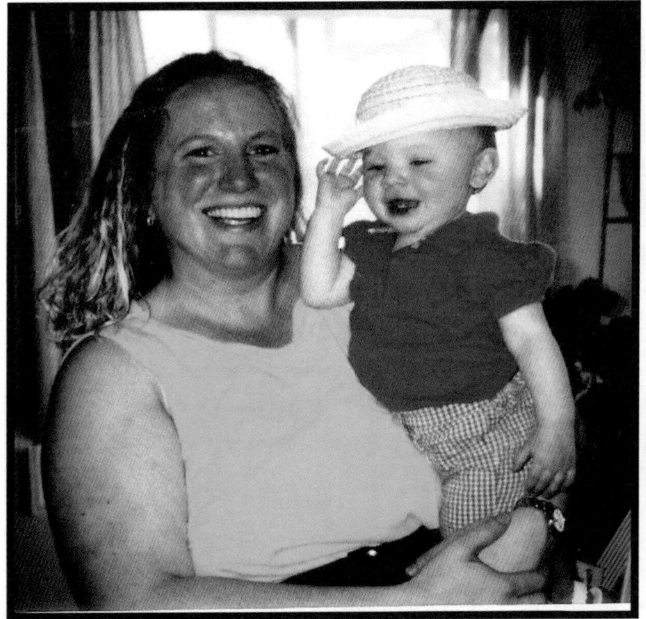

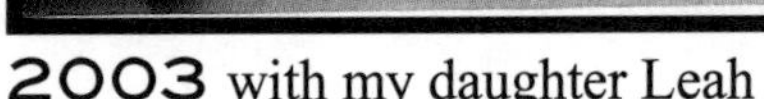

2003 with my daughter Leah

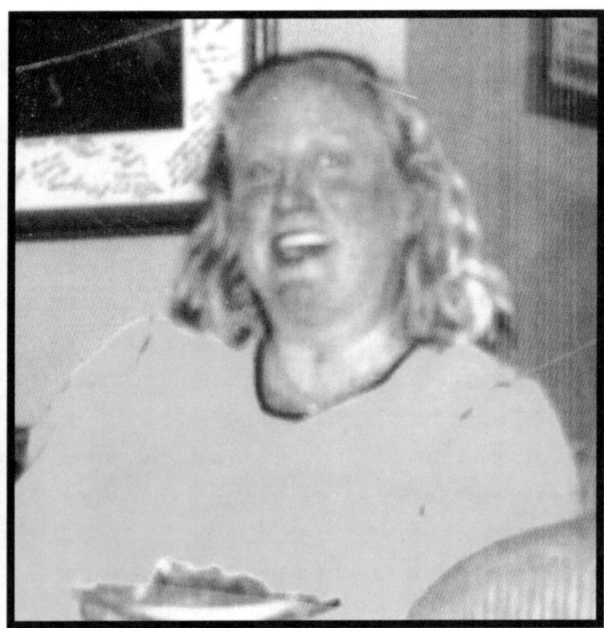

2006 (**'ish**) Me with pie.

WHERE THERE IS NO STRUGGLE, THERE IS NO STRENGTH
—OPRAH WINFREY

BTW, Oprah started out as a newscaster and completely sucked at it. So she tried the talk show thing. BA-BAM!

FIT HAPPENS

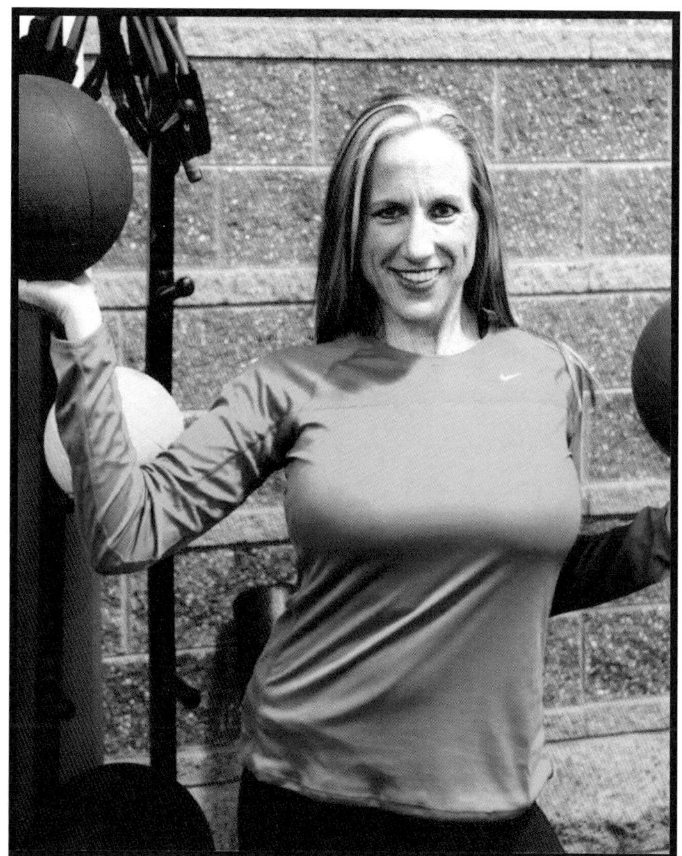

2012

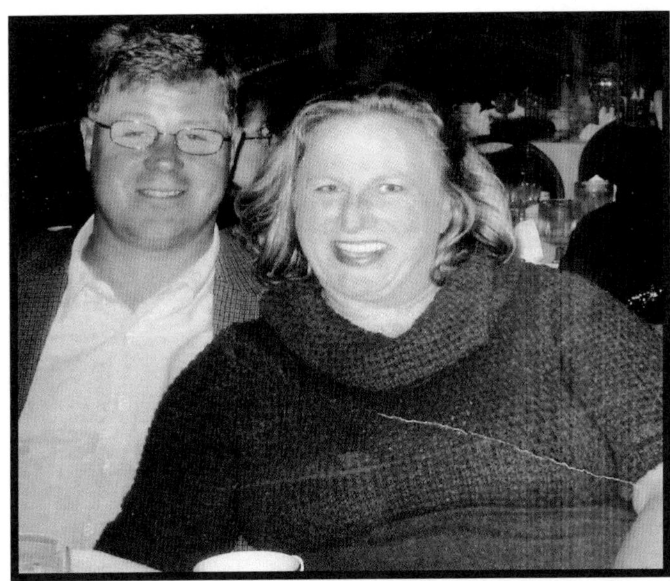

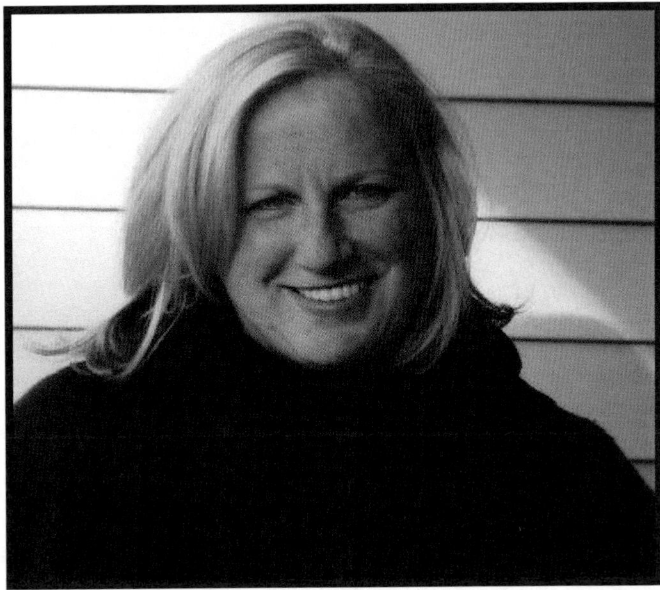

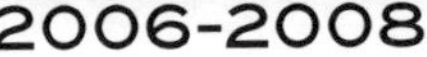

2006-2008

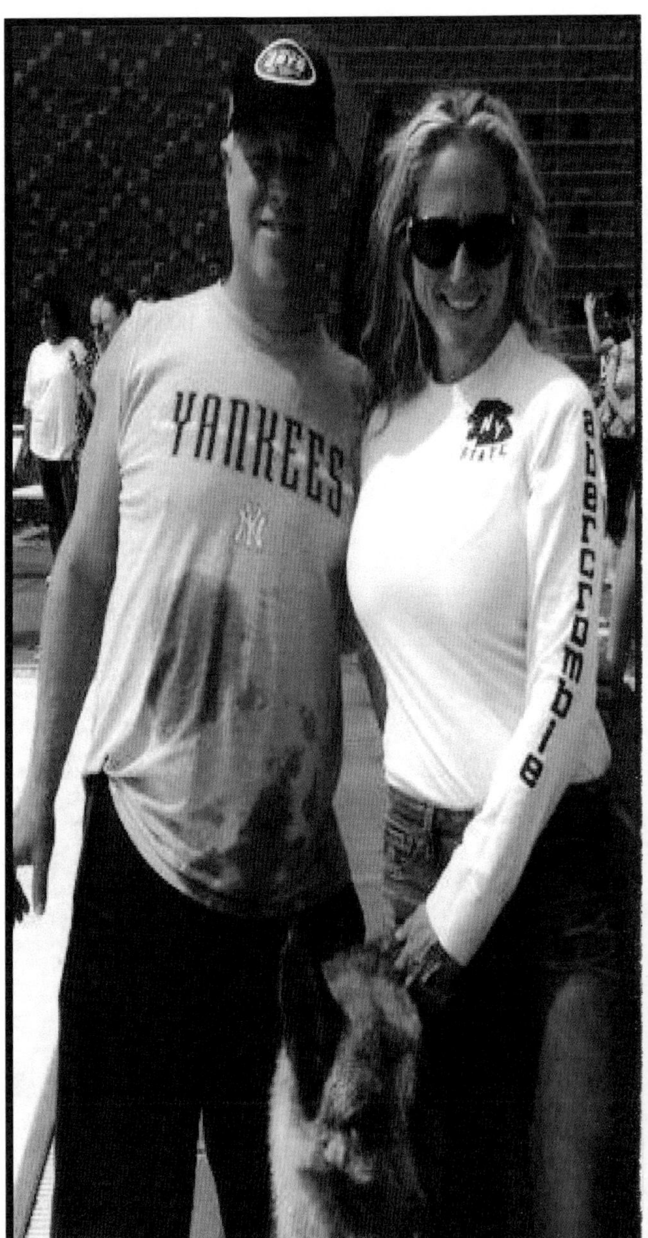

2011

BACK IN BLACK!

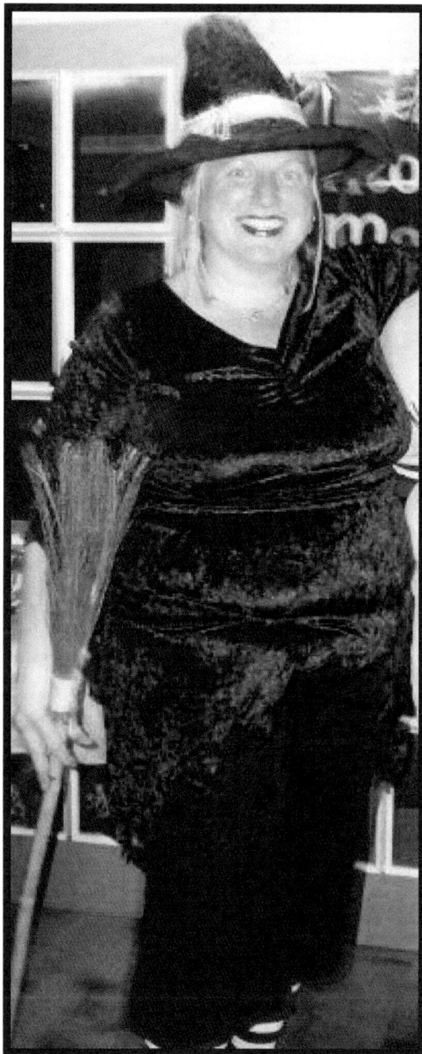

HALLOWEEN 2006

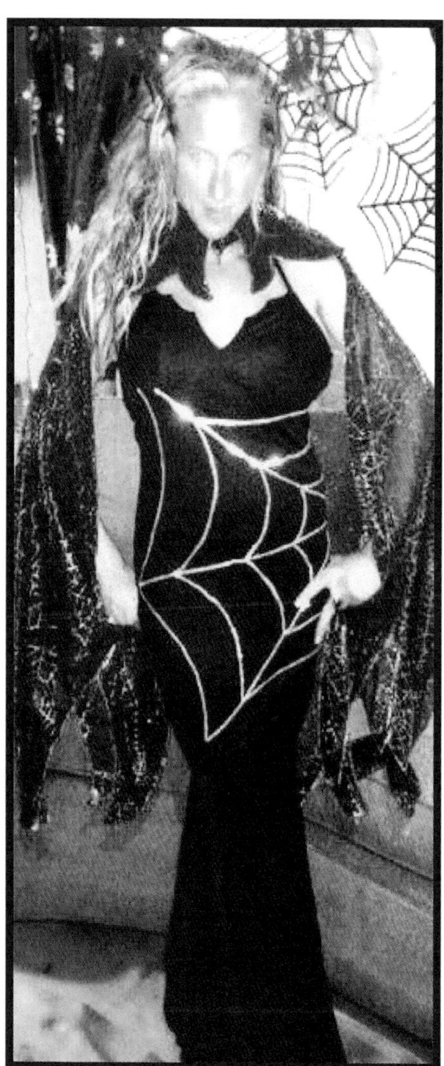

HALLOWEEN 2011

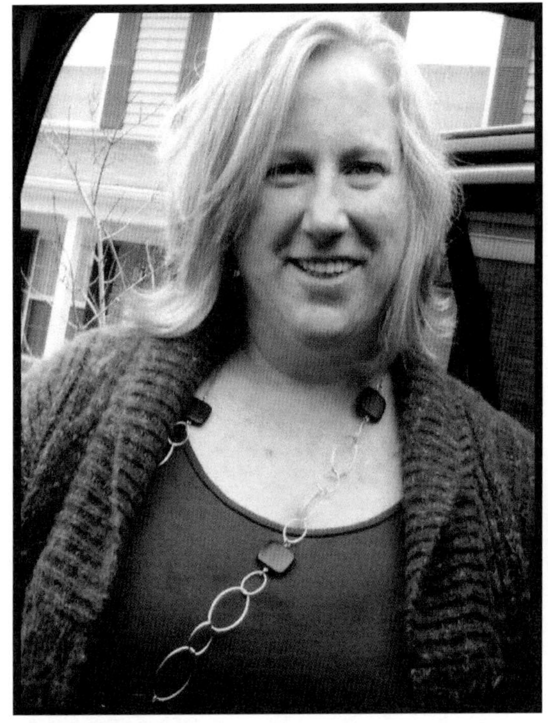

2008

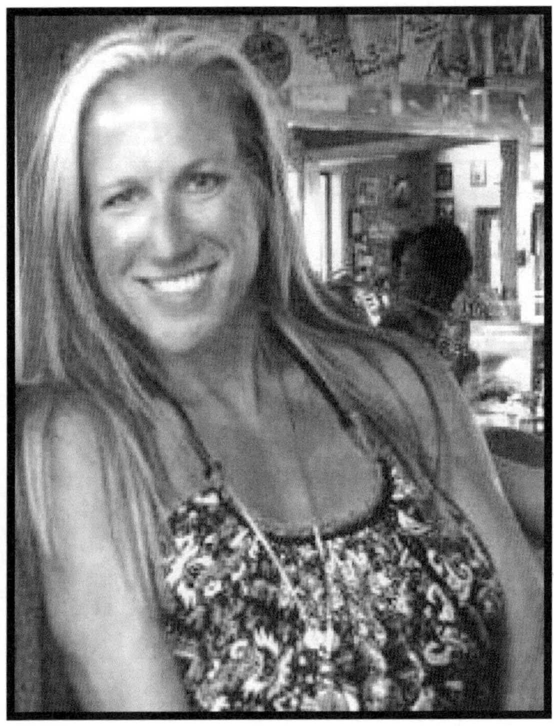

2012

IT'S JUST AS EASY TO PUT ON A SASSY T-SHIRT AS IT IS TO PUT ON A CRAPPY ONE. IT'S ESPECIALLY EASY WHEN YOU FEEL GOOD ABOUT YOURSELF FROM THE INSIDE OUT.

YOU GO GIRL!

NEVER give up on YOU. NEVER.

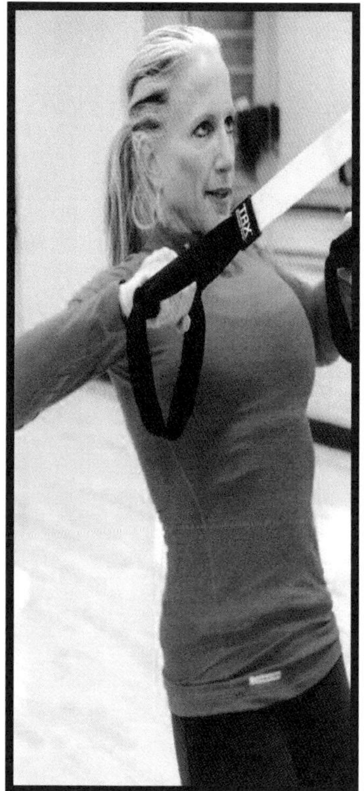

OCTOBER 2012

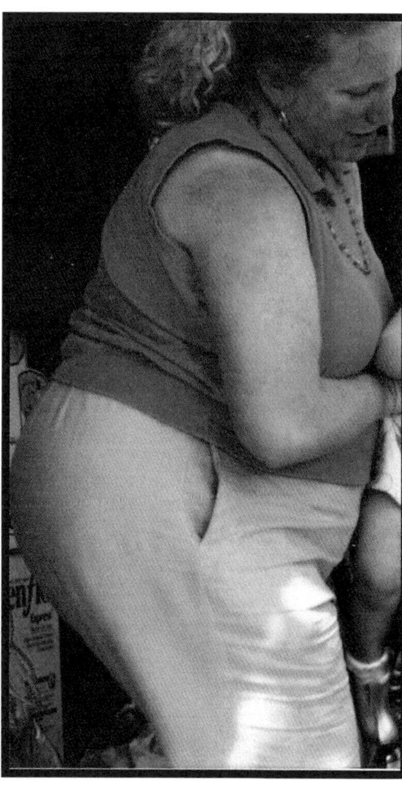

2003 padonka donking

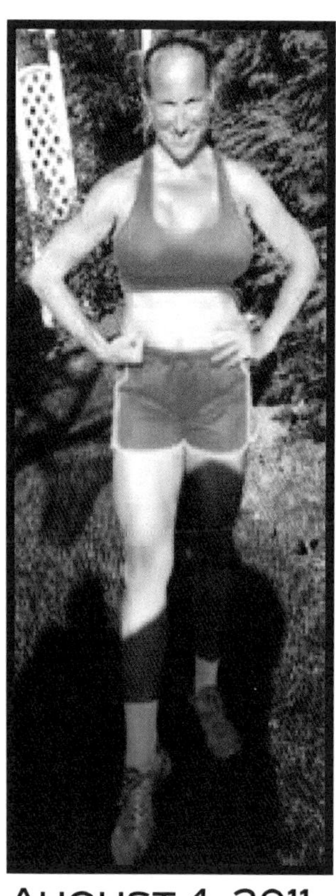

AUGUST 4, 2011,
2yrs. Post-op

I'VE FAILED OVER AND OVER AND OVER AGAIN IN MY LIFE,
AND THAT'S WHY I SUCCEED
—MICHAEL JORDAN

It's people like MJ that help me see failure in a whole new light. BTW, can I call you MJ?

"IT IS NEVER TOO LATE TO BE WHAT YOU MIGHT HAVE BEEN."
—GEORGE ELIOT

WHEN YOU ARE BEHIND, NEVER GIVE UP.
WHEN YOU ARE AHEAD, NEVER LET UP!

GET YOUR STRONG ON!

"START BY DOING WHAT'S NECESSARY; THEN DO WHAT'S POSSIBLE; AND SUDDENLY YOU ARE DOING THE IMPOSSIBLE."

--ST. FRANCIS OF ASSISI

CLEAN VERSION:
-ASK YOUR DOCTOR IF GETTING OFF YOUR BUTT IS RIGHT FOR YOU-

EXPLICIT VERSION:
-ASK YOUR DOCTOR IF GETTING OFF YOUR A$$ IS RIGHT FOR YOU-

-NO MATTER HOW YOU ACHIEVE YOUR WEIGHT LOSS, YOU WON'T BE ABLE TO MAINTAIN IT UNLESS YOU ROCK THE LIFESTYLE CHANGES-

-MAKE TODAY RIDICULOUSLY AMAZING-
(EVEN IF "TODAY" IS A COMPLETE WASTE OF MAKEUP)

<u>NEVER</u> GIVE UP ON YOU. <u>NEVER</u>.

- YOU MISS 100% OF THE SHOTS YOU NEVER TAKE-
(YOU MIGHT STILL MISS THEM ANYWAY, BUT AT LEAST YOU TOOK THEM)

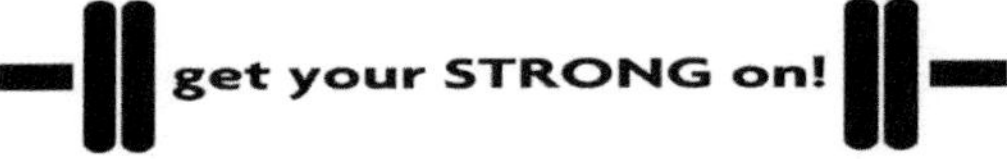

-STRONG IS THE NEW SKINNY-

-SKINNY IS OVERRATED! SO GET YOUR STRONG ON!-

-CHANGE OCCURS WHEN INSPIRATION AND
MOTIVATION MEET PERSPIRATION-

-STRETCH YOURSELF BEFORE YOU WRECK YOURSELF-
-JOLYNN WRIGHT

When it comes to exercise, eating right (or anything really)...
-YOU DON'T HAVE TO LOVE IT...
YOU JUST DON'T HAVE TO HATE IT-

WHEN ALL ELSE FAILS...GO PEE

-OLD HABITS DIE HARD,
OLD THINKING DIES EVEN HARDER-

-STICKTOITIVENESS:
STAYING ON IT LIKE WHITE ON RICE;
HAVING A KUNG-FU GRIP ON YOUR GOAL-

-WHEN IN DOUBT, I ASK MYSELF "WHAT WOULD
300-POUND ME DO?" ONCE I HAVE THE ANSWER,
I RUN LIKE THE DICKENS IN THE OTHER DIRECTION-

-MY BEST THINKING GOT ME TO 300 POUNDS,
NOT MY BEST ACTIONS-

-NO MATTER HOW SLOW YOU GO, YOU'RE STILL LAPPING
THE GUY ON THE COUCH-

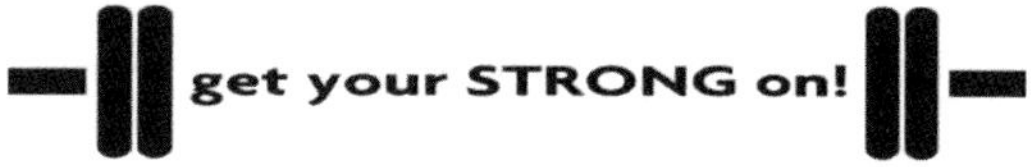

Just in case I wake up stupid… I like to keep some definitions handy.

avoid— to stay the heck away from

change— the act, process, or result of making or becoming different (by doing the complete opposite of what I used to do)

hope – a chance or likelihood for something desired, something wished for…basically—I gotta shot!

hunker down— to prepare to stay in a place or position for a long time, usually in order to achieve something. Then once you are all hunkered down…don't budge.

insanity— (insert 300-pound me picture here) repeating the same patterns of behavior and expecting different results. Worse than insanity is indifference…repeating the same patterns of behavior and not giving a you-know-what about what happens.

inspire— to move or guide by divine influence, to move (someone) to act, create, or feel emotions: arouse, to cause something to be created or done. To give a glimmer of hope.

never— not ever, at no time, not to any extent or in any way

strong— (insert 150-pound me picture here)
healthy, having powerful action or effect

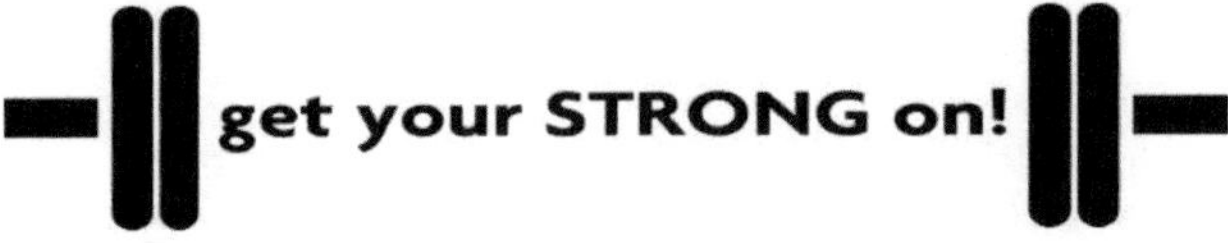

I'm certainly not the boss of you or anything...but here are some tips on how I ROCK the lifestyle changes (and by "rock" I mean recommit to them on a daily basis)

DO's
DO dare to prepare (pack your lunch the night before, and bust out the travel cooler)
DO have your gym clothes ready the night before, and always keep an extra set in your car
DO ask for help when you need it (and we all need it), and remember childcare at the gym equals WINGMAN!
DO get off the couch
DO cheer yourself on…YOU GO GUUUUUUUUUUUUURRRRRRRRRRRRRRL!
DO assemble an "A-team" to support you
DO try new things, but don't play with firecrackers, I mean food
DO kick "fake hungry" to the curb, and if you see "fake skinny" kick her B-hind
DO have self-awareness and hunker down
DO remember that awareness without action gets you bupkis
DO remember how well your best thinking has worked for you in the past
DO remember the definition of insanity and the trap door of indifference
DO make time for YOU (not just in leap years, but regularly)
DO say NO to the second carb serving and SALADIZE instead
DO use a salad plate (instead of eating off of a serving platter)
DO repeat what you eat (take the guess work out of "what you *feel* like eating")
DO get help setting realistic goals
DO have a plan at social gatherings and places where boxes of candy and cookies multiply like rabbits…then channel your inner sticktoitiveness

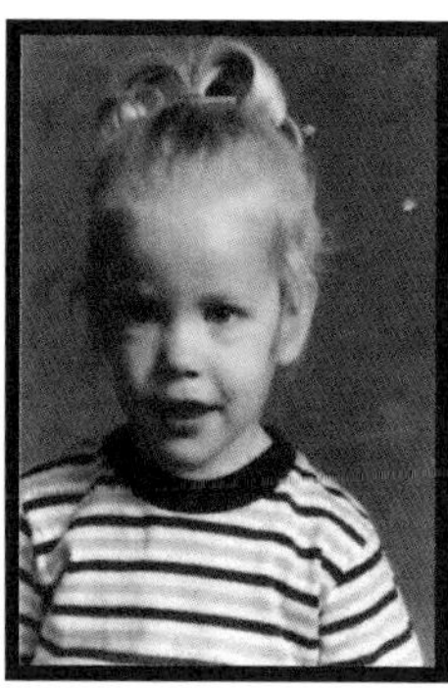

DO keep a photo of yourself as a child with you at all times…and treat yourself like you would treat that child
DO have a blast (or if you're not there yet…be willing to have a blast at some point)

DON'Ts
DON'T be a knucklehead…seek direction from trained professionals, and access resources in your community—(FYI the Y offers wellness coaching to start you off…for FREE! And, the PT rates are very reasonable)
DON'T grab and go and continue to grow
DON'T scarf and barf
DON'T be ashamed of who you are
DON'T get sucked into negative thinking (yours or anyone else's)
DON'T be unfair and compare yourself to others, (especially supermodels)
DON'T hang out where the food smells kruh-mazing more than you have to
DON'T give up on YOU
DON'T destroy pleasantly plump photos of yourself…you just may need them some day

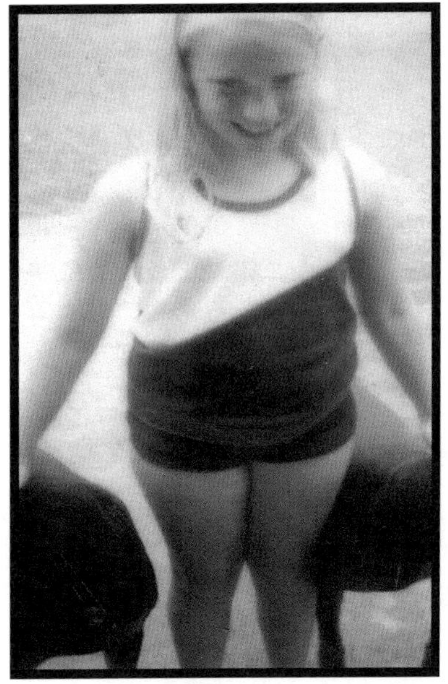

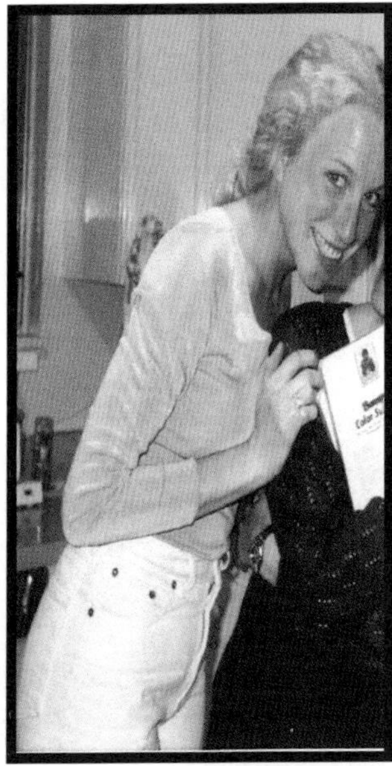

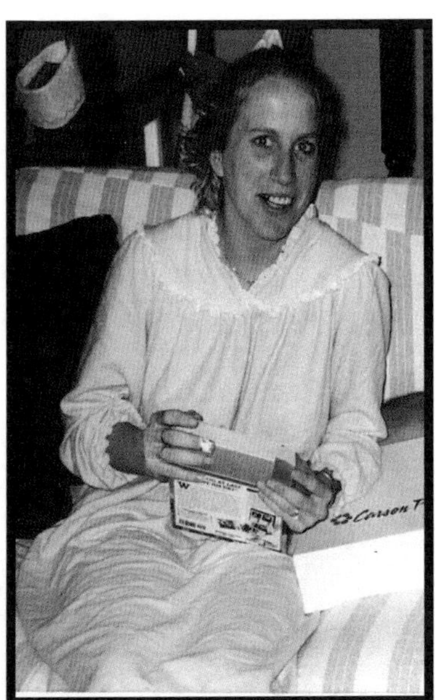

FROM CHUNKY... TO FAKE SKINNY...

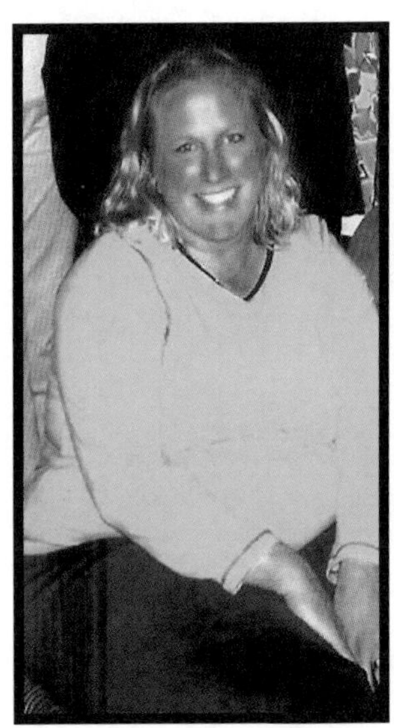

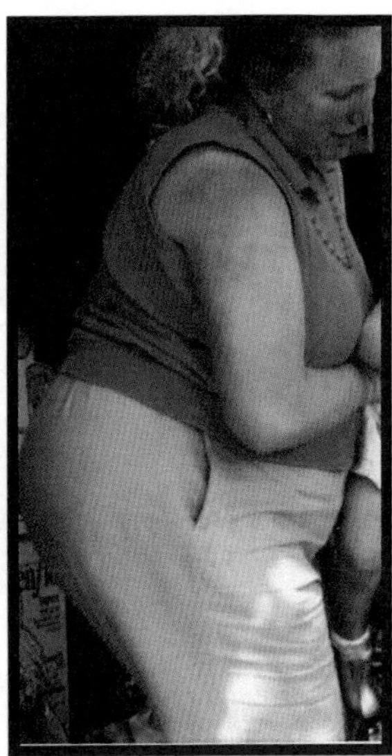

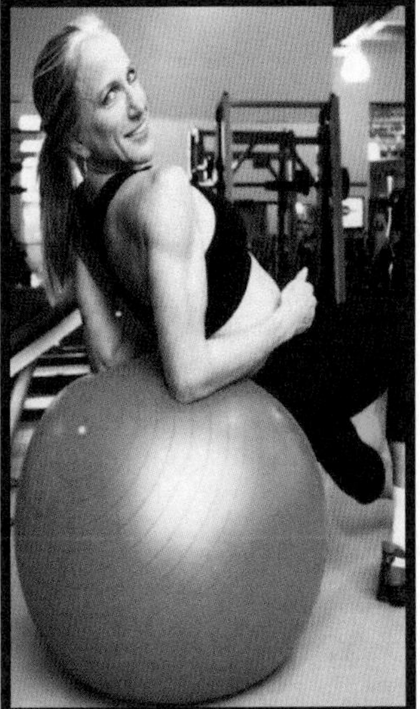

TO INDIFFERENCE... TO STRONG!

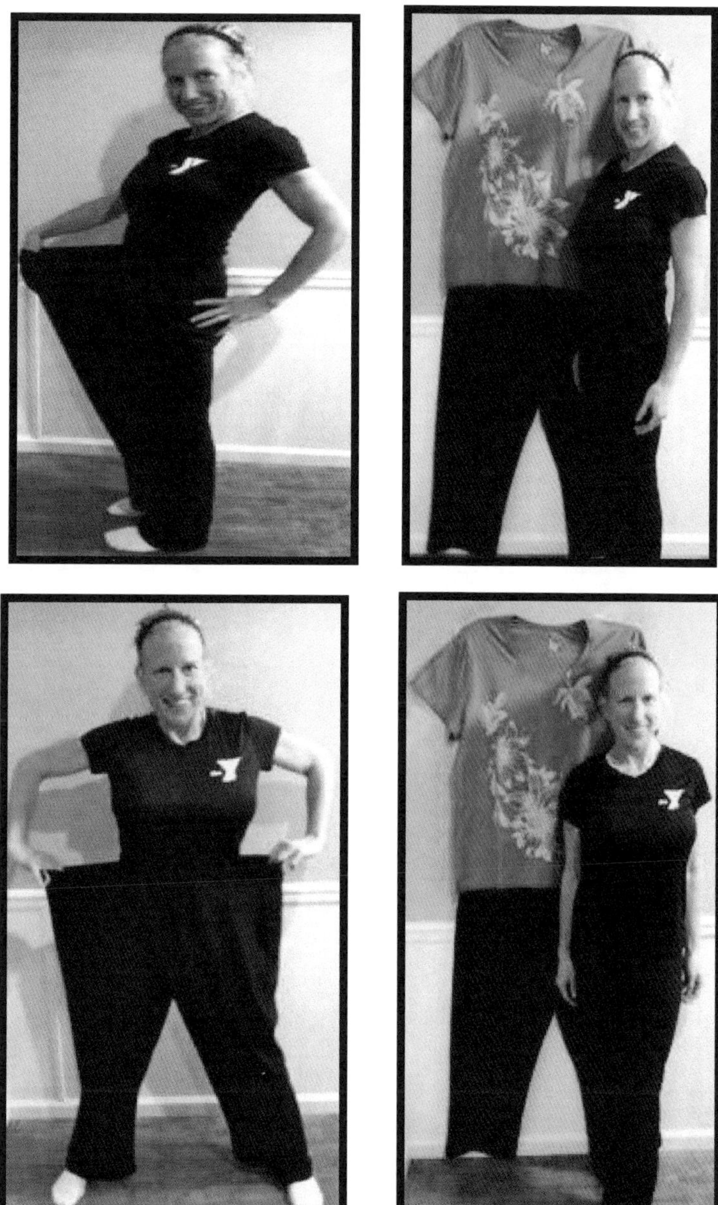

I've been bossy pants, fancy pants, silly pants, and sassy pants, but this is a first…

standing in my pants!

Very bulimic in 1993'ish…"take the damn picture already so I can go throw up".

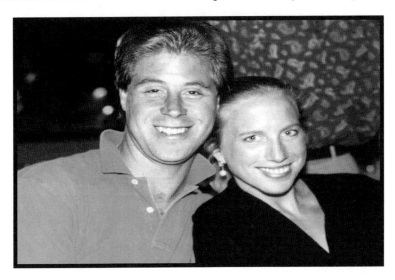

July 2012 at an event without abusing food. (BTW, that's not the same shirt on my husband. Not only did he get a new one, but he spared us all the flipped up collar this time around.

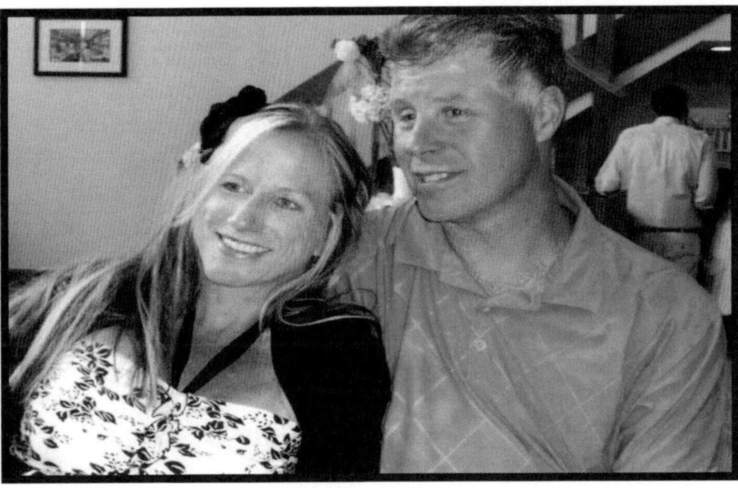

DESCRIBE THIS PHOTO:

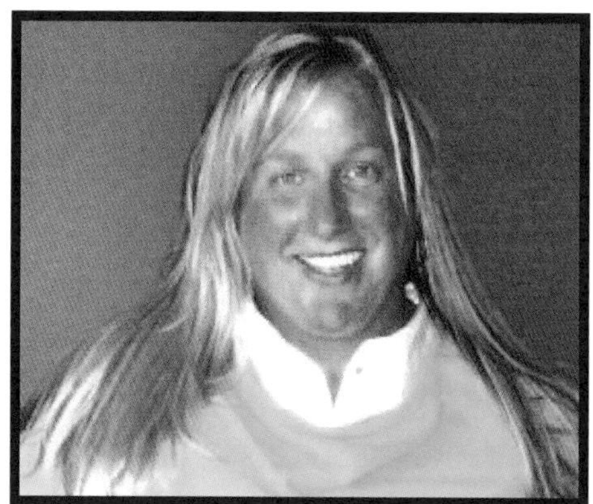

Miserable, out of breath, sweaty, hot (but not "hot-to-trot" hot), and my favorite…Professor Sherman Klump's long lost sister from another mother. For those of you who were still watching Barney or weren't alive yet, see The Nutty Professor 1996).

existing at 300 pounds

DESCRIBE THIS PHOTO:

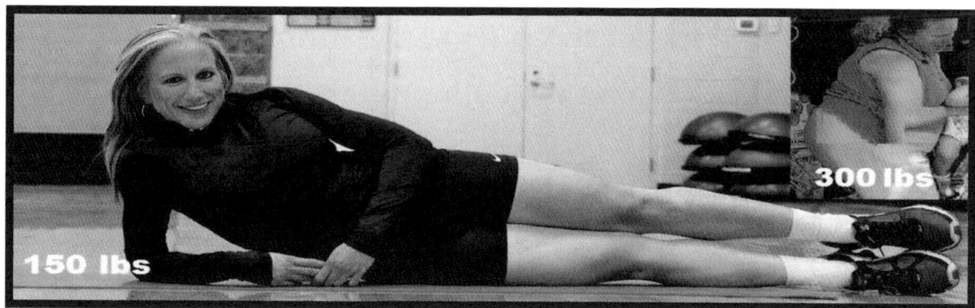

Really?, Seriously?, AYFKM?, Holy Moly!, Kruh-mazing, Holy crappits!, Magnifitastic, Smexy, Terrifical, Shut the front door! (and the back door too), You go girl! ("gurrrl").

A woman who got her life back.

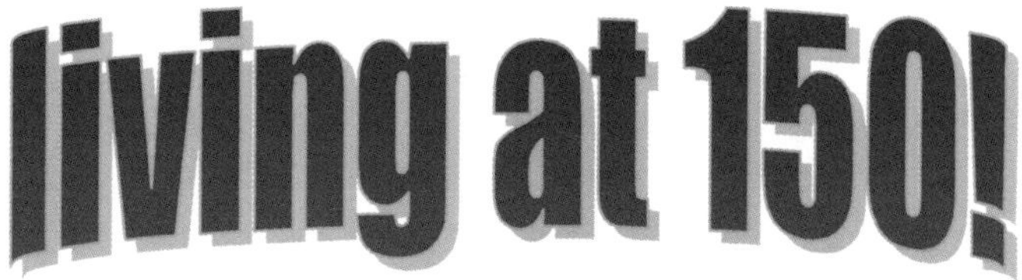

Acknowledgements

This is the part where I thank my agent and fancy pants publisher. Since I don't have either of those (yet) I will thank whoever they will (hopefully) be in advance. (Thanks guys, you rock). Now let's write some books! Have your people call my people, and by "my people" I pretty much mean me, unless one of my kids answers the phone.

But seriously, thanks a bazillion to the following people, places and things:
The Fishers YMCA for amazing support cheering me along the entire way
The "A" Team - Dr. Brenda Cacucci, Dr. Neil Wanee, Dr. John Aker, Dr. Muhammad T. Munir
and Matthew G. Newmann, A.C.S.M., C.P.T, M.S. Kinesiology
St. Vincent Bariatric Center of Excellence
Stephanie, Denise, Tommalisa, Kimberly & Tiffany for showing a girl how to shake it
McDonald's on 131st Street in Fishers, IN for a fine cup of Joe for $1.08
(and the booth I took hostage many a morning writing this book)
To all of the people in this world that throw a blind squirrel a nut once in a while
Webster's Dictionary (just because)

And I always save the best for last:
Rabbis Bernie King, Richard Steinberg, Brett Krichiver, Nadia Siritsky, Paula Winnig, and Cantors Arie Shikler, Irving Green, and Janice Roger for reminding me of so many wonderful things
Mom, Aunt Didi, Brandy and my BFF Jennifer for believing in me. Debra for going above and beyond.
Ray, for never giving up on me and loving me through a very long decade of dog years
And, (in order of appearance in this world) Davis, Leah, and Halle who are the silliest,
most amazing kiddos a mother ship could ever hope to care for

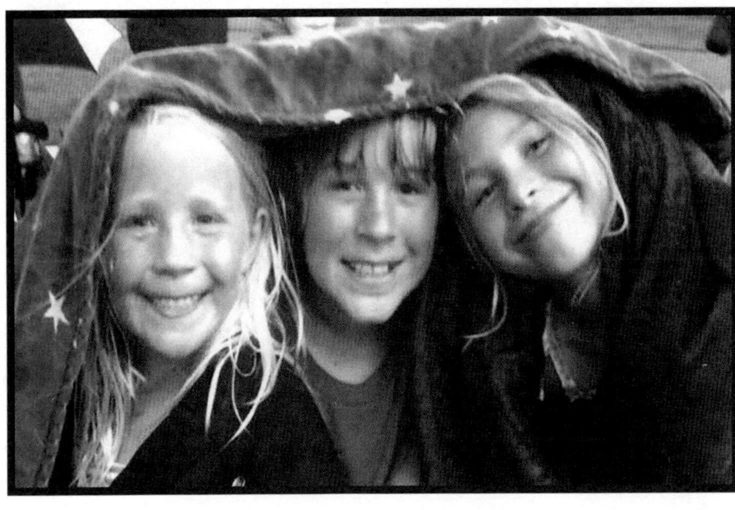

If I could fast forward to my 100th birthday, I would offer my
40-something-year-old self the following snippets of truth:

Hindsight has the advantage of being just that…HINDSIGHT. As Webster's likes to break it down, "the understanding of something only after it has happened." Well, since I'm 100 and you're not, LISTEN UP. There are so many things to get lost with in life's day-to-day grind. Do your best to look beyond that drudgery. Enjoy the humans around you. Cherish laughter and moments. Drop perfection at the door, and for the love of God, don't worry how clean your house is. You're not going to look back and wish you had spent more time mopping the floor (trust me on that one, sister). Appreciate health and wellbeing, and ask for help when you need it. Don't yell at the little people that look up to you (or anyone for that matter). Remember that learning is life-long and there is value in failure. If you don't believe me, just ask Michael Jordan who got cut from his high school basketball team, or Oprah who was fired from her first TV news gig. Don't be indifferent to the plight of others, or yourself for that matter. Always have a German Shepherd named Sam, and maybe a neurotic cat or two. Keep love and life in the forefront, and make sure you care for YOU. And one more thing...it's pretty funny that your name is Robanne Robin.

THE END

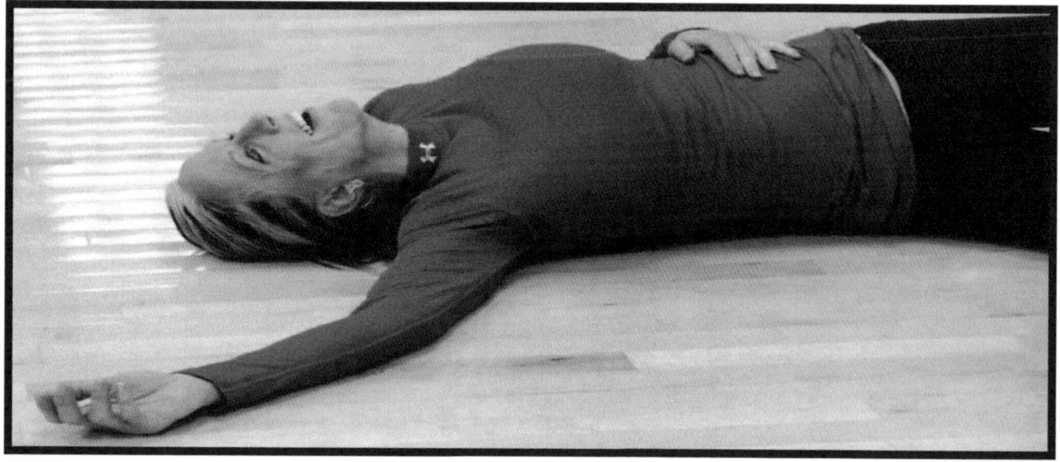

Note to self: Much like losing weight and keeping it off, writing a book is hellaciously HARD.

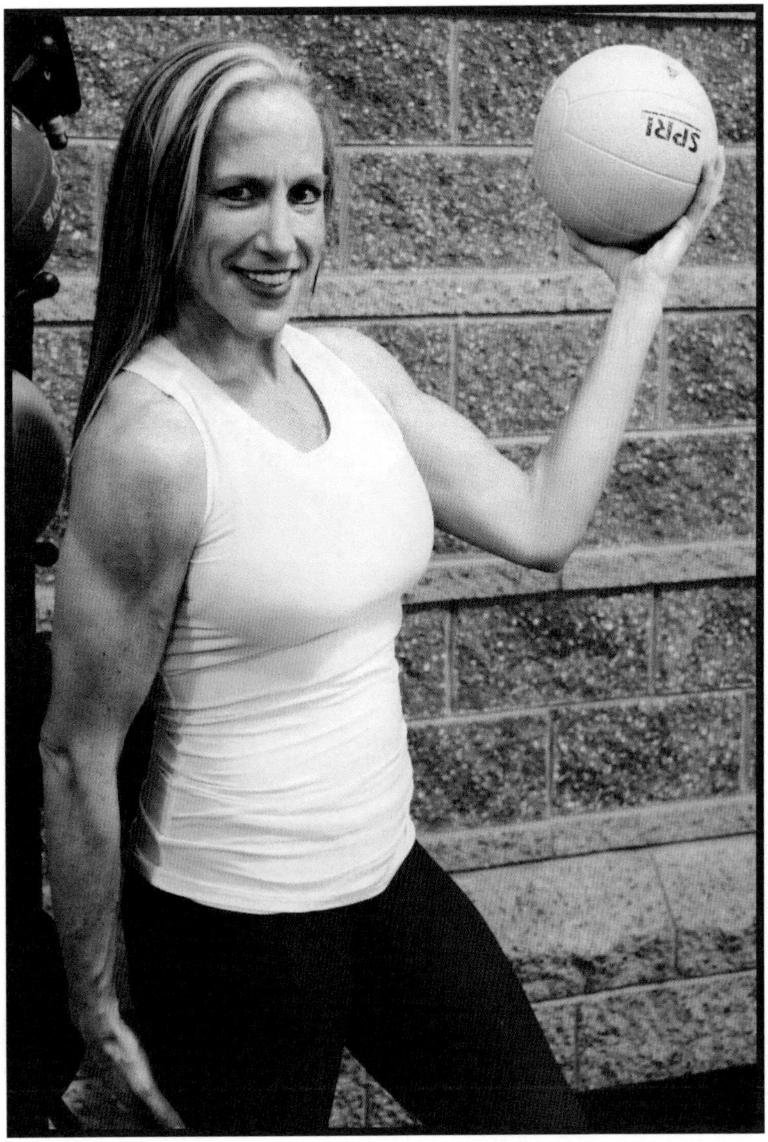

Other books coming in 2013-2014 by Robanne Robin:

Get Your STRONG On!
ISBN 978-0-9885755-4-7

SAG
ISBN 978-0-9885755-2-3

Saladize Me!
ISBN 978-0-9885755-7-8

Eat. Train. Live.
ISBN 978-0-9885755-8-5

Diary of a Minivan Mom
ISBN 978-0-9885755-6-1

Butterfly
ISBN 978-0-9885755-9-2

Get Your STRONG On!, LLC
P.O. Box 50985
Indianapolis, IN 46256-0985
getyourstrongon@gmail.com

www.getyourstrongon.net

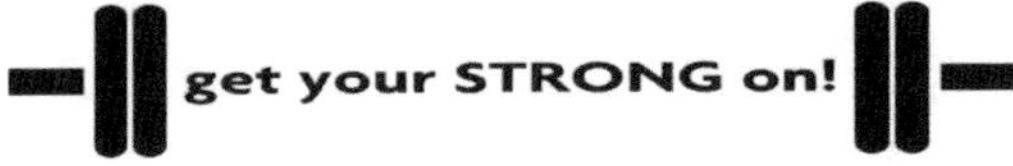

These t-shirts and others available on our website

**Ask your Doctor
If Getting off your Butt
is Right for you**

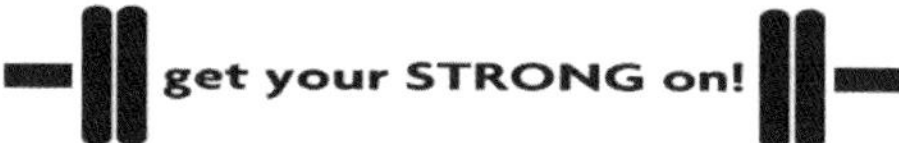

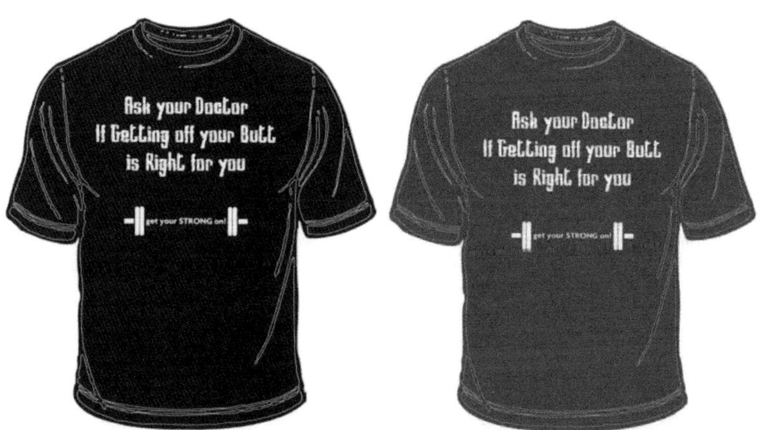

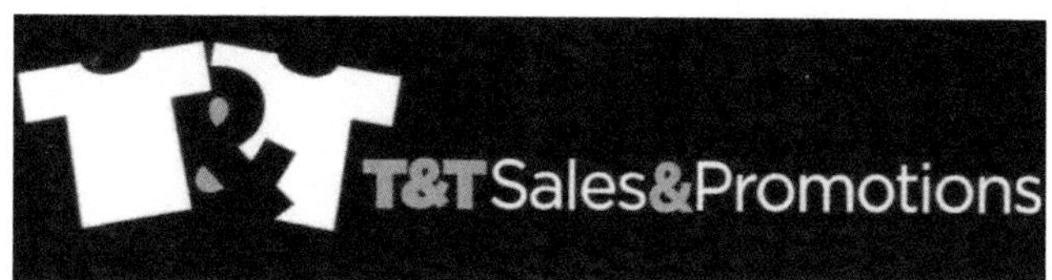

15320 Herriman Boulevard
Noblesville, Indiana 46060
Tel: 317.774.7106
Fax: 317.774.8035
tntsalespromo.com

Learn more about getting your STRONG on at www.getyourstrongon.net

STRONG
is the new skinny

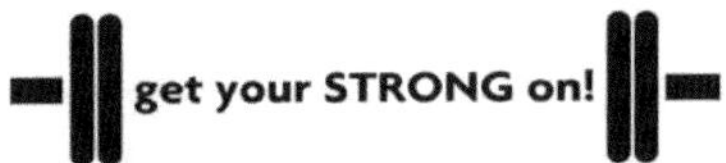

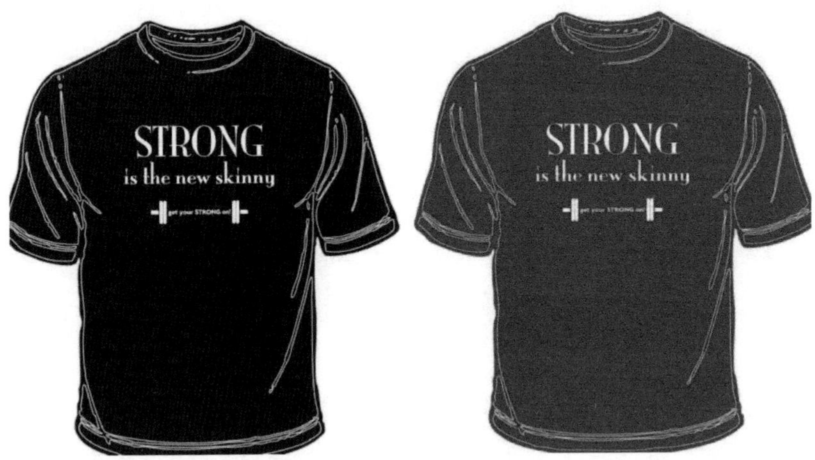

Learn more about getting your STRONG on at www.getyourstrongon.net

No matter how
slow you go,
you are *still*
lapping the guy
on the couch.

get your STRONG on!

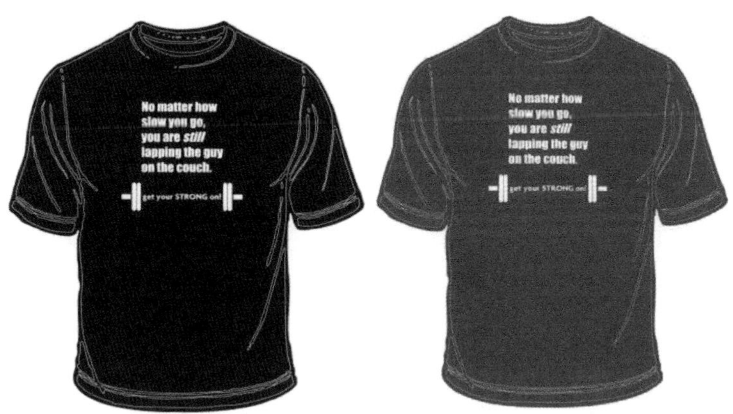

Learn more about getting your STRONG on at www.getyourstrongon.net

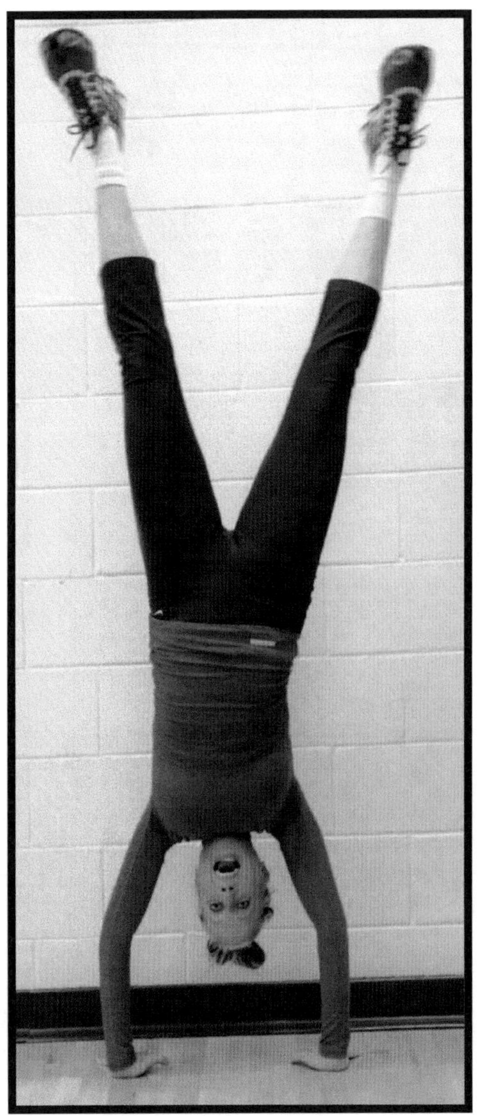

LIVE WELL, LOVE MUCH, LAUGH OFTEN

(and do a handstand once in a while)

ROBANNE ROBIN (in order of experience) is a wife, mother of 3, Registered Nurse, certified Hip Hop Hustle instructor, and author. She has battled eating disorders all of her life including childhood obesity, anorexia, bulimia, and morbid obesity as an adult. At age 37 Robanne was facing major health issues including high blood pressure and diabetes. After two trips to the ER with a pulse over 200 she knew she had to make some serious lifestyle changes, or risk continued health problems. On August 4, 2009, Robanne had lap-roux-en-Y gastric bypass surgery and has since lost half of her body weight. She has gone from weighing 300 pounds to 150. After almost giving up on herself, Robanne sought medical help that has saved her life. Through seeking help and putting in the hard work to make major lifestyle changes, she has turned a lifelong struggle with weight and eating disorders into a platform to motivate and inspire others. She now lives an active lifestyle and has launched books and inspirational projects. Robanne works with bariatric patients to motivate them to be successful. Additionally, her passion is to encourage kids to re-think being skinny, and shift their focus to being STRONG and fit. She works to inspire and motivate anyone who struggles with eating disorders and weight issues. Robanne shows her audiences that STRONG is the new SKINNY and above all shares the message that anyone can make changes. Robanne earned a B.A. in Communications from California State University Fullerton, and a B.S. in Nursing from Indiana University School of Nursing. The best "degree" Robanne earns on a daily basis is her fitness by getting her STRONG on five times a week at the YMCA in Fishers, Indiana. And…she finally got her first Hip Hop instructor gig at the Fishers Y.

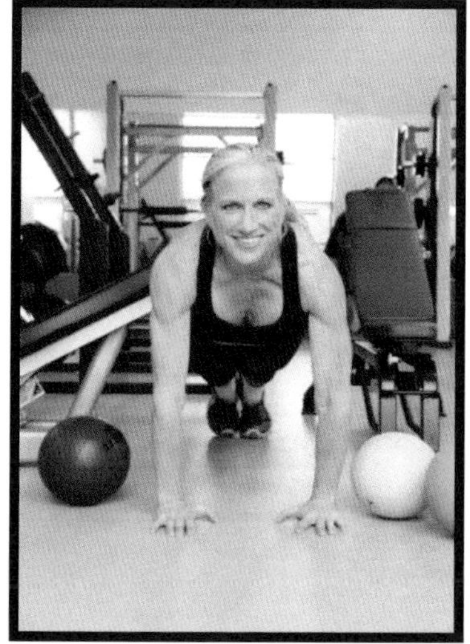

When you are behind, **NEVER** give up...
and when you are ahead **NEVER** let up.

NEVER give up on YOU. **NEVER**. She almost did, and look what's happening to her.
Learn more about our message of health and wellbeing at www.getyourstrongon.net

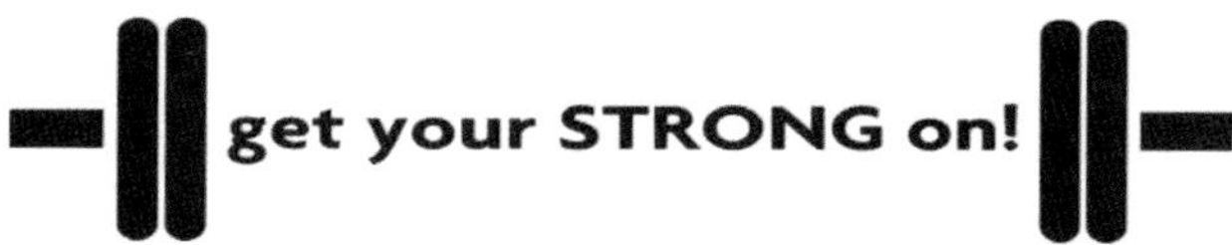

Made in the USA
Charleston, SC
20 December 2012